T0323750

"This book is essential reading for anyone who wants to understand how the brain works to enable learning, and what this means for educational practice. Rogers and Thomas provide an authoritative but accessible introduction to the incipient field of educational neuroscience, bringing to life the latest evidence from brain science and its implications for learning with engaging case studies and exemplars, and debunking 'neuromyths' along the way. A must for teachers and other educationalists committed to exploring the evidence on what works in teaching and learning – and to understanding *why* it works."

Professor Becky Francis, *Chief Executive of the Education Endowment Foundation (EEF)*

"Here is a trustworthy guide to what every teacher needs to know about the brain. It explains findings from neuroscience in down-to-earth language and discusses what goes on in the brain when we are learning to read or to do maths, when we need to remember, make friends, think, and multitask. It also serves as a primer of research methods and carefully considers what can and cannot be translated into practice This enlightening book is a joy to read and will help teachers to make learning more effective."

Dame Uta Frith, *Emeritus Professor of Cognitive Development, Institute of Cognitive Neuroscience, University College London (UCL)*

EDUCATIONAL NEUROSCIENCE

THE BASICS

Educational Neuroscience: The Basics is an engaging introduction to this emerging, interdisciplinary field. It explains how the brain works and its priorities for learning, and shows how educational neuroscience, when combined with existing knowledge of human and social psychology, and with teacher expertise, can improve outcomes for students.

Cathy Rogers and Michael S. C. Thomas reveal how neuroscientific evidence is forcing us to question our assumptions about how our brains learn and what this means for education. The chapters in this vital volume step through the brain's priorities: processing senses and moving our bodies, emotional processing, and the difficult job of dealing with other people. It unpacks the tricky tasks of thinking and learning, considering how memory works and the many systems involved in learning. It draws this all together to offer guidance for effective classroom practice, current and future. Chapter features include key issues for special educational needs and neurodiversity, case studies of novel interventions, debunking of common neuromyths, and guidance for teachers on how to evaluate their own practice.

This book is a compact, lively introductory text for students of psychology, neuroscience and education and courses where these disciplines interconnect. It will also be essential reading for educational professionals, including teachers, heads, educational advisors and the many industry bodies who govern and train them, as well as anyone interested in the fascinating story of how we learn.

Cathy Rogers completed her PhD in Educational Neuroscience at Birkbeck, University of London, after many years spent producing science television shows. Her research interests are diverse and include the effects of digital technologies on brain development and the neuroscience of adult literacy. Her primary area of interest is in the brain basis of creativity.

Michael S. C. Thomas is Director of the Centre for Educational Neuroscience at Birkbeck, University of London. His research interests are in the translation of research between neuroscience and education, establishing new transdisciplinary accounts in the learning sciences, and developing practical applications within education. He is a Chartered Psychologist, Fellow of the British Psychological Society, Fellow of the US Association for Psychological Science, and Senior Fellow of the Higher Education Academy.

The Basics

The Basics is a highly successful series of accessible guidebooks which provide an overview of the fundamental principles of a subject area in a jargon-free and undaunting format.

Intended for students approaching a subject for the first time, the books both introduce the essentials of a subject and provide an ideal springboard for further study. With over 50 titles spanning subjects from artificial intelligence (AI) to women's studies, *The Basics* are an ideal starting point for students seeking to understand a subject area.

Each text comes with recommendations for further study and gradually introduces the complexities and nuances within a subject.

For a full list of titles in this series, please visit www.routledge.com/The-Basics/book-series/B

EDUCATIONAL NEUROSCIENCE

THE BASICS

Cathy Rogers and Michael S. C. Thomas

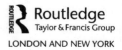
Routledge
Taylor & Francis Group

LONDON AND NEW YORK

Cover image: monkeybusinessimages/iStock via Getty Images

First published 2023
by Routledge
4 Park Square, Milton Park, Abingdon, Oxon OX14 4RN

and by Routledge
605 Third Avenue, New York, NY 10158

Routledge is an imprint of the Taylor & Francis Group, an informa business

British Library Cataloguing-in-Publication Data
A catalogue record for this book is available from the British Library

ISBN: 978-1-032-02887-3 (hbk)
ISBN: 978-1-032-02855-2 (pbk)
ISBN: 978-1-003-18564-2 (ebk)

DOI: 10.4324/9781003185642

Typeset in Bembo
by Taylor & Francis Books

Cartoons © Pier Helm

CONTENTS

ILLUSTRATIONS

FIGURES

With sincere thanks to Piers Helm for the cartoon illustrations

TABLE

BOXES

WHY DO WE NEED EDUCATIONAL NEUROSCIENCE?

INTRODUCTION

Psychologists have come up with many proposals for how learning might work. Teachers have a huge amount of experience of what seems to work. The aim for educational neuroscience is to figure out how learning *actually works*, in the real-life, messy, biological organ that is the brain. By understanding the real mechanisms of learning, we can optimise all the systems geared to improving it, that is: teach.

There are many unanswered questions about human behaviour. Psychology has tried hard to answer them. But the trouble with psychology is it relies on looking at behaviour from the outside – and looks can be deceiving. In particular, things that seem like one thing from the outside are actually many things inside the brain. Take someone saying, 'I'll keep that in mind': it sounds like a single thing. The reality though is that there are many systems all over the brain that keep account of recent brain activity for possible future use. They each rely on a different cocktail of ingredients, which vary depending on context and content, to work well. 'Keeping something in mind' sounds simple but in the brain it's actually pretty complicated.

In this chapter, we introduce the core ideas of educational neuroscience and explain the need for this approach. We also give an honest assessment of where we are on the educational neuroscience journey; bluntly, barely out of the gates. And we touch on why there has sometimes been reluctance to include neuroscience within a multidisciplinary approach to education.

DOI: 10.4324/9781003185642-1

THE POTENTIAL OF EDUCATIONAL NEUROSCIENCE

> I think there is a huge prize waiting to be claimed by teachers. By collecting better evidence about what works best and establishing a culture where this evidence is used as a matter of routine, we can improve outcomes for children, and increase professional independence.
>
> – Ben Goldacre, 2013

Nearly everything that teachers do works (Hattie, 2008; Tokuhama-Espinosa, 2014). Some things work really well. Other things work a bit. There are quite a few things where we don't have the evidence to say too much yet. If we can gear more teaching to those things which we know work really well, we will improve effectiveness, that is, we will help more children learn better.

In the past few decades, medical practice has undergone a quiet cultural and scientific revolution. Before the revolution, best practice was often determined by experience, status or charisma – your family doctor knows best, the god-like consultant knows *everything*. After the revolution – that is, now – best practice is instead founded on scientific evaluation of what works best for improving outcomes for patients. Medical practice is served by a huge research and development industry which investigates better drugs and more effective treatments. The work of the GP is supported by the medical research industry, by diagnostic guidance, by NICE guidelines.[1] Put like this, it is hard to argue against wanting the same for our children's education. And that, in essence, is the goal of educational neuroscience: to bring evidence-based practice to education, with how we educate children being informed by what we know gives them the best outcomes, in turn, informed by what we know about how learning works in the brain.

'Evidence-based' is not the same as 'neuroscience-based'. And while educational neuroscience embraces any approach that uses scientific evidence of outcomes – that is, findings that robustly demonstrate A works better than B – it also wants to ask, '*How* does it work?' Neuroscience, in other words, want to take things a step further by studying what actually happens in the brain. This isn't necessarily the same as we might conclude by looking from the outside.

1   National Institute for Health and Care Excellence.

BOX 1.1 TOOLS OF NEUROSCIENCE

Brain scans are an important tool of neuroscience. These colourful pictures of brains are a wonder of science and seem to be every-where – but they can sometimes be misleading. They can give the impression that things are more certain than they are, particularly when writers describe parts of the brain 'lighting up' when people do or think a particular thing. It all sounds so neat: cause and effect, case closed. In reality, evidence from brain scans is rather messier. Let's roll up our sleeves.

A common type of neuroimaging is the fMRI (functional mag-netic resonance imaging) scan. The basis for measurement is the fact that blood carrying oxygen has different magnetic properties from blood that isn't carrying oxygen. We know that active tissue requires oxygenated blood, so by extrapolation we can look at areas which are using more or less oxygenated blood. So the measure is quite indirect: not the chemical or electrical activity of neurons, but the metabolic requirements of areas of neurons. This has many implications, but one big one concerns speed: blood flows a lot more slowly than neurons fire (the average cortical neuron fires between 1 and 30 times a second (it's variable); the brain blood oxygen signal is also variable but can take around 10 seconds to reach its peak) – so fMRI is better at saying *where* in the brain something is happening than precisely *when*. Another important consideration is that fMRI does not measure brain activity by itself but *in relation to* another brain activity; a brain scan is a *comparison*, for example, between what is happening in the brain when someone is trying to come up with alternative uses for a paperclip versus when they are just looking at a paperclip and thinking how to describe it. The fMRI results are the difference in brain activity between these two tasks – which theoretically determines the spe-cific areas that are crucial to (in this case) generating an idea.

Another neuroscience tool is electroencephalography (EEG), which measures electrical activity in the brain through receptors that pick up tiny electrical signals through the skull (it involves wearing one of those chic caps). An advantage is that EEG is measuring direct neural activity – so it can be quite specific about timing, but since skull position only maps roughly to brain area, it is not so good on positioning. The opposite of fMRI, EEG is better on *when* than *where*.

Both techniques – and many similar ones used in the lab – (magnetoencephalography (MEG) – which uses the property of the magnetic field the brain emits or functional near-infrared spectroscopy (fNIRS), which uses the extent to which the brain's tissues absorb light shone through them) – involve highly artificial settings, obviously very far from the classroom. The latest cutting-edge technology is trying to make these techniques more portable, indeed wearable, so that scientists can observe the brain's operation as people go about their everyday lives, or students pay attention (or don't) to the teacher in a classroom. Perhaps they will even allow us to observe how the teacher's and students' brains are synchronised.

Educational neuroscience draws on many sources of evidence – neuroimaging tools, animal experiments, single neuron studies, computational models, eye tracking, behavioural psychology experiments, genetic studies, quantitative and qualitative classroom assessments and more. Neuroscience is not just brain imaging, it's a set of different methods to answer the question, 'how does the brain work?' The key is that, if there is converging evidence from many different sources that point to similar findings, it gives much greater confidence that effects are real – and that they operate not just in the confines of the lab but also out in the real world.

Let's take an example, drawn from how children learn about scientific ideas. From the day they are born, children wake up and experience the sun coming up and going down. It's quite reasonable for them to deduce from this that the sun goes around the Earth – it's obvious! They've seen it with their own eyes! Then one day they go to school and are taught that, no – the Earth goes around the sun. What? This seems crazy! It defies their perceptions! But with a bit of support and good teaching, they can learn this new, true version of events.

How is this change of knowledge brought about in the brain? The traditional view was that the earlier (incorrect) knowledge is replaced, overwritten by the later (correct) knowledge. But evidence from scanning the brain – so-called neuroimaging (see more in Box 1.1 'Tools of neuroscience') – has shown that it's more complicated: brain networks involved in *inhibiting* or blocking the old knowledge are also highly activated when people are arriving at the new knowledge. In other words, *both* sets of knowledge continue to exist in the brain. To get to the correct knowledge, a part of the brain must 'Sshhh' the part of the brain chiming in with its old, naïve knowledge, covering its mouth for long enough for the new knowledge to chirp up with the right answer (Brookman-Byrne et al., 2018; Houdé et al., 2000; Masson et al., 2014).

This is pretty surprising stuff. But it has potentially wide implications, because there are lots of things that children learn at school which might run counter to their prior knowledge. In biology, they learn about fish and mammals – then along come dolphins. In maths, they learn that higher numbers are bigger (6>3) but then negative numbers and fractions appear to change the game: -6 is smaller than -3, a sixth is smaller than a third. They learn in physics that heavy and light objects fall at the same rate. Eh? That doesn't chime with what they've seen in the real world, where the hammer plummets and the feather wafts to the ground. Their powers of inhibition need to be working on overdrive. This is just one example of something we have learned with the help of neuroscience. It now forms the basis of an intervention designed to improve outcomes in science (see Box 1.2).

BOX 1.2 CASE STUDY: 'STOP AND THINK'

How do children learn new concepts? The traditional view of conceptual change was that new learned theories replace old ones: once a child learns that the Earth rotates around the sun, their previous theory (based on their experience of seeing the sun move) that the sun rotates around the Earth, would be overwritten. Recent evidence from adults suggests something more surprising: that these old, incorrect theories remain stored in the brain; often we still need them to drive our perceptual expectations such as where to look for the sun in the sky. But in an educational context, we need inhibitory control to suppress them in order to reach the newer, correct theories. The naïve incorrect theory is more familiar and automatic; the new theory needs time and deliberate suppression of the old theory to be actively retrieved.

The *UnLocke* intervention (funded by the Wellcome Trust and the Educational Endowment Trust in the UK) trained children to engage this analytic system and inhibit their automatic system. Over several lessons, children completed a computerised game, comprised of science and maths curriculum content, which encouraged them to inhibit an initial response, in favour of a more delayed and reflective correct response, under the ruse of helping contestants in a gameshow. The content was focused on some of the many counter-intuitive concepts that exist in science and maths and the intervention was delivered as part of normal science and maths lessons.

The results of the large, randomised control trial were independently analysed, and revealed that over the course of a single term, children in the 'Stop and Think' game intervention group made on average the equivalent of one additional month's progress in maths and two additional months' progress in science compared to children in the control group. Research is ongoing, particularly to test the feasibility of making the intervention more widely available. See https://www.unlocke.org/

EMPOWERING TEACHERS

Many people want to have a say in education. Teachers are probably heartily fed up with being told what they should be doing – and of ever shifting changes in education policy. Evidence-based practice should empower teachers because scientific evidence doesn't wax and wane every 5 years. It provides a solid base from which teachers can use their skills and expertise to build the best lessons for their students. Teachers, like doctors, are craftspeople with personal expertise built up from years of learning from experience, both their own and that of their peers. Coupling all this with the solid grounding of evidence of what works best overall, they have the expertise to modify and adapt interventions to the unique needs of their individual students. Educational neuroscience is a truly interdisciplinary endeavour, bringing together the combined expertise of teachers, psychologists, neuroscientists, and developmental scientists, all focused on improving outcomes for students.

Teachers broadly seem to welcome the idea of this sort of collaboration. A survey of teachers by the Wellcome Trust (Simmonds, 2014) found a high level of interest in neuroscience. Although more than 60 per cent said they knew 'just a little' about how the brain works, 82 per cent said that they were interested in knowing more and 54 per cent had looked up information on the brain in the past four weeks. These findings suggest an unmet appetite for neuroscience knowledge.

In the same survey, teachers were also asked about their current use of some specific approaches which were (accurately or inaccurately) portrayed as based on neuroscience evidence. These were approaches based on learning styles, left/right brain distinctions, Brain Gym® and biofeedback. A large number of teachers used such approaches in their classrooms – the highest percentage (76 per cent) using learning styles approaches and the lowest percentage (1 per cent) using biofeedback, which most teachers (67 per cent) had not heard of. Some 16 per cent were using Brain Gym® and 18 per cent were using approaches based on left brain/right brain distinctions.

These results are slightly less encouraging. They highlight the fact that there are many tools and products available which boast brain-level claims and appear to present a compelling case – but without supporting evidence. For learning styles, there is even evidence that using approaches which target interventions to children's preferred learning styles (e.g., using visual materials for 'visual learners', kinaesthetic materials for 'kinaesthetic learners') can actually be harmful if used strictly. This is because there is strong evidence that students learn better when multiple modalities are offered rather than just one. Undue focus on one modality can mean that children miss out on opportunities to fully develop their skills in other domains.

This leads us to a tricky problem. Namely, that teacher enthusiasm – and corporate hunger to develop and use neuroscience-based applications – are out of step with the actual science. In reality, there are very few currently available, systematically evidence-based neuroscience approaches available for the classroom. So while it is encouraging that there is willingness to embrace new approaches, it is important that they are in fact effective ones.

There are other barriers to the interdisciplinary ambition to have neuroscientists, psychologists and teachers working together (Churches et al., 2017). These include:

- *Different goals.* Neuroscience is a natural science in its adolescent stage of development. It still has gaping holes in its understanding of detailed brain function and is still primarily concerned with building a basic science research base about the detailed workings of the brain. Teaching is a practical endeavour geared to daily improving outcomes for children.
- *Different levels of description.* Neuroscience tools include many levels of analysis, from studying genes to single neurons to brain networks to whole brains. Educational investigations begin at the level of the whole student and go all the way up to the level of society and culture.
- *Different words.* Sometimes things get lost in translation between the very different languages and jargon of different professions. Accurate translation takes expertise, commitment and time.

TEETHING ISSUES

The educational neuroscience project has its detractors. There are some who argue that brain-based evidence is just too far from classroom practice to be useful and that the field is exploiting popular fascination with brain scans. Others say that neuroscience methods are too imprecise and that the field is still at too early a stage to be able to properly interpret findings, never mind translate them into intervention recommendations. Still others complain that neuroscience doesn't bring anything new to the table, but really just constitutes a relabelling exercise, replacing psychological terms with the names of brain structures. Some see neuroscientists as just another group of people telling teachers what to do. And there is the ongoing issue of tackling 'neuromyths' – highly infectious misconceptions about the brain.

Some humility is needed. There is a huge amount of work to be done to build meaningful and productive collaborations between all the parties involved – to get teachers to lead research rather than have it arrive from labs, to work harder at translating basic science into potential application and much more. This work is under way (Hobbiss et al., 2019; Tokuhama-Espinosa, 2014). But it will take time. Just as the cultural change to evidence-based medicine took many decades, so too will a similar move in education.

Educational neuroscience certainly doesn't claim that neuroscience will improve education on its own. Rather, it aims to bring together evidence from different descriptive levels to converge on the most effective proposals for the classroom. Educational neuroscientists are not blinded by the lights of an MRI scan. They understand that working in partnership is the key to success. To give an example, the Wellcome Trust and the Education Endowment Foundation (EEF) funded six projects under the educational neuroscience banner which were all interventions designed to improve school outcomes in different areas. Many were based on neural as well as psychological evidence and involved teachers not only in implementation but in some cases in development and design. The resulting interventions, which took place in existing school settings, were tested on both behavioural (psychological) outcomes – did the children perform better at GCSE, for example? – as well as using lab studies to look at whether there was evidence of the predicted brain-level changes (that is, whether the theory of what would elicit change was reflected in the brain) and qualitative evidence from teachers about their experience of the intervention (was the approach practically achievable and a desirable alternative?). It is not one or other, but all types of evidence, combined (Howard-Jones et al., 2016; Sigman et al., 2014; Thomas et al., 2020).

YOU WOULDN'T TELL A BABY TO RUN

Education and learning are constrained by the functional workings of the brain. In the following chapters, we will go back to the basics of what the brain is, where it has come from, evolutionarily speaking, and what its priorities are. It might be surprising that the type of learning children experience in schools is very far from its main goal (its most fundamental aim is to keep us alive, see Figure 1.1) – which is why learning can be pretty hard. (If you're thinking our low/high priority is upside down in Figure 1.1, there is method to our madness!

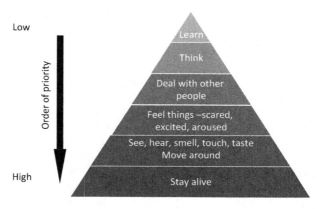

Figure 1.1 The brain's hierarchy of priorities

See Figure 1.2) New cultural acquisitions – things like using tools, playing music, reading or doing maths – can only be added to our repertoire by fitting into our brain's pre-existing architecture, which came about because of its ability to perform much more basic functions. We don't start playing music because of a new 'music' add-on, or learn to read because of a literacy plug-in. Taking on these new skills means co-opting and sometimes contorting the brain to do something it wasn't designed to do. Things work the way they do in large part because of our evolutionary history and the flexibility of our neural systems to adapt to experience. Not because they have been perfectly designed for that job.

We will go into more detail about this hierarchy in the coming chapters, but for now the important point is that *school learning is not what the brain was designed to do.* Indeed, if we set out to design something to optimise learning, we would almost certainly not end up with the brain! We will see in Chapter 6 that learning involves at least eight different systems in the brain – some connected with memory, some with staying on track with the learning task, some based on rewards, some based on long-term practice. Learning is one of the hardest things for the brain to do, both in terms of energy and in the coordination of all these systems. One implication of this, a pretty big one for teachers, is that people will only do it – learn – if their internal cost/benefit analysis tells them it is worthwhile. Think of it like this: running is harder than walking – but if you really want to get somewhere on time, then you will choose to make the extra effort to run. The same goes for learning. Some things require more energy/effort but if you really want to get somewhere, you will be prepared to spend that energy. The question is really, 'How much do you want to get there?'

Any system with so many moving parts also has many potential points of failure, or weakness – and diagnosing and understanding those are an important part of the project to better understand learning.

Thinking of the brain in this way also makes it clear that if students' more basic needs are not met, then learning cannot possibly be optimised. By 'more basic' we mean everything from really basic, such as being properly nourished and getting enough sleep, through to less obviously basic such as not feeling intimidated by a teacher or being emotionally engaged enough to pay attention. Such observations will not be news to teachers or to psychologists. In fact, the prioritisation hierarchy presented in Figure 1.1 has many similarities with Maslow's well-known hierarchy of needs (see Figure 1.2), which is getting on for a century old.

The difference is that, where these needs have typically been presented in terms of differentiating 'physical' from 'social' from

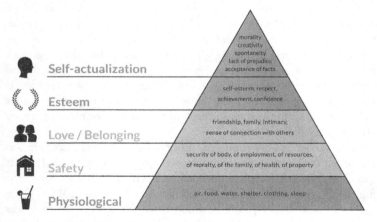

Figure 1.2 Maslow's hierarchy of needs, 1943

'mental' needs, at the level of the brain, there is no such neat compartmentalisation. There is no brain/mind/body division. There is no separating out the 'purely emotional' from the 'purely cognitive'. That's just not how brains work.

Certain things are possible for the brain and certain things aren't. We wouldn't ask a baby to run because its brain and body do not yet have the capacity to execute that movement. It feels obvious to us. As we understand other aspects of how the brain works, other new things become equally obvious. For example, asking 12-year-olds to maintain concentration for the full duration of a double period of geography on a Friday afternoon is very likely to exceed their attentional thresholds. Or if maths seems scary to a child, perhaps reinforced by a teacher's subtle anxiety in presenting the material, it is no wonder that the child's brain will be more concerned with plans to escape the situation than with learning what these new hieroglyphics mean.

HOW CAN NEUROSCIENCE HELP?

Neuroscience helps us to understand why things happen. Sometimes this understanding might shine a light on new things, and sometimes – particularly in these early days of the educational neuroscience journey – it might enrich our understanding of things we already know from other sources of evidence. For example, healthy meals have long been a tenet of good educational practice, for many reasons, including providing energy for the cognitive effort of learning and playing, ensuring healthy physical growth and development, and reducing sickness. Neuroscience has a particular interest in nutrition since the brain is by far the biggest consumer of energy of all the organs in the body, typically gobbling up about 20 per cent of all our intake.

Beyond basic energy count, the specifics of nutritional intake are also important for learning. For example, we now know that high-fat diets can cause NMDA receptors on brain cells which are critical for learning, to become desensitised (Valladolid-Acebes et al., 2012). These findings could be of particular importance for students from lower socioeconomic groups, whose nutritional options are often more limited (Hackman et al., 2010). Based on this and other evidence, the

Education Endowment Foundation (EEF) toolkit[2] recommends school breakfast clubs as a low-cost, high-impact route to improving outcomes for students – both for the direct benefits of providing healthy meals at the start of the day, and indirect ones that arise through improved attendance, punctuality and achievement (Grantham-McGregor, 2005). More work is under way on specific nutritional interventions, such as exploring whether giving Vitamin D, Omega-3 or other dietary supplements has a positive effect on learning.

In a similar vein, the benefits of physical exercise extend to many aspects of student well-being, and few would question the wisdom of students exercising regularly. But from the point of view of maximising learning, *how regularly* and *for how long* might be optimal? We know that physical exercise benefits the brain through diverse mechanisms – from generalised effects such as improving blood flow, lowering stress hormones and stimulating growth factors, to specific effects such as enhancing neural growth in the hippocampus, a brain area key to memory formation. Specific research in this area is likely to prove useful – but also highlights the lengthy journey from animal studies to lab studies with people, to studies in the real world, with many new questions being thrown up by research findings en route. For example, a recent study looking at the effects of physical activity found that it was more strongly associated with greater *emotional* regulation in younger children (7-year-olds) and with greater *behavioural* regulation in older children (11-year-olds) (Vasilopoulos & Ellefson, 2021). Such findings illustrate the difficulty of meeting a demand for simple, specific, practical recommendations, such as the optimal exercise schedule for students of different ages (Erickson et al., 2011).

Good sleep is another basic requirement for effective learning. What do we mean by 'good sleep'? Current recommendations from the National Sleep Foundation are for 9–11 hours of sleep for 6–13-year-olds, 8–10 hours for teens and 7–9 hours for adults.[3] But even these are guides just to quantity; sleep research shows that quality of sleep, and the proportions of REM and slow wave sleep are also important. One of the key features of sleep is that the way that sleep establishes memories simply would not be compatible

2   See https://educationendowmentfoundation.org.uk/education-evidence/teaching-learning-toolkit
3   See https://www.thensf.org/

with the brain's normal awake mode of operation. Wait, what? It's a bit of a brain twister – but consolidation of memories – that is, the process which firms up new, shaky memories by connecting them to pre-existing long-term memories – happens by running those memories through the same networks that were involved when the experiences were originally processed. If this happened in the awake brain, it could cause huge confusion – hallucinations, double memory formation, all sorts. The waking brain works well for encoding memories. The sleeping brain works well for consolidating them. It's a fundamental principle of how brains work in all mammals that the two should be kept apart.

We know that significant sleep benefits come from an 8-hour night of sleep. Perhaps more surprising is that many of those benefits are also seen after shorter naps of just 1 or 2 hours (Diekelmann & Born, 2010). This has led some to propose (Sigman et al., 2014) that naps, already a feature of many early year childcare providers, should be facilitated within the school setting. Other more dramatic interventions have been proposed which involve changing school start times (that is, starting school later) for teenagers, since changes to circadian rhythms in adolescence make early mornings particularly challenging for them. There is something of a cautionary tale here, one that nods towards the multiple influences that shape everyday educational practices; a study designed by neuroscientists based on good evidence of the changed sleep needs of adolescents proposed the introduction of later school start times for A-level students. They had not fully considered the huge practical implications for schools and parents of such a change – not just class timetables, but also coach services, lunch services, after school clubs and more – which in the end made the project untenable. The project was redeveloped, this time led by teachers, into one geared to improving the quality of teen sleep, through better sleep education of teens, such as not using tablets or phones in the dark last thing at night, because the blue light disrupts the onset and quality of sleep (Illingworth et al., 2020; Mireku et al., 2019).

While neuroscience evidence has added to our existing understanding of these basic, organism-level needs of nutrition, exercise and sleep, it has also had more direct effects. One striking example has been in improving outcomes for deaf children. Universal hearing screening of new-borns, based on the development of tools to detect oto-acoustic emissions, has meant that interventions can now start much earlier. Traditional detection using psychological tests was only possible for infants already several months old. Children who receive cochlear implants earlier (usually before the age of 3) acquire vocabulary and develop speech faster, and show better reading comprehension than age-matched peers who received implants at a later age.

This is a different example of how neuroscience evidence is relevant for learning outcomes, one that does not rest on dialogue between researchers and teachers. It is included to show the breadth of what educational neuroscience might include and as a signal of what might come, as knowledge improves, and early detection is enabled for other learning-relevant difficulties.

CHANGING MINDS

Teachers are involved every day in manipulating the human brain. In fact, teachers are really the only people whose specific job it is to change the connections between neurons in their students' brains. Sounds almost scary put like that! It also makes you think – imagine designing a sock without knowledge of a foot (Hart, 1999; Sousa, 2011). And while this is not the book where you will learn about anatomical names or the biochemistry of synapses (though do check out the Resources section for suggestions of where you can find that kind of thing), there are some basic governing principles which it *is* important to know. We will be revisiting these throughout book.

So first, let's talk about plasticity. It's key to learning, but what exactly is it? Well, most simply, it is the process by which the connections between neurons are changed in response to stimulation from the environment. There are some pretty important things to know about plasticity:

- The brain remains plastic right through life – from the womb, right into old age – it is evolution's way of allowing brains to adapt to the bodies and environments they find themselves in.
- It's thanks to plasticity that people can recover from some forms of brain damage, by the brain changing its connections in response.

- Plasticity is a feature of *all* learning processes, whether that's playing the piano, kicking a football, learning a language, or remembering what happened yesterday.
- Without plasticity we would be unable to learn new things or form any new memories.
- The degree of plasticity is not constant. It can be reduced as a result of stress, ageing and injury, and increased through sleep, exercise and learning.

WHAT DOES ALTERING NEURON CONNECTIONS HAVE TO DO WITH LEARNING?

Well, a lot. Here's an analogy of how we might think about learning. Imagine that you are at the edge of a forest and you want to get to the other side. The forest is thick with trees, brambles and dense undergrowth. The first time you try to go through, it will take a lot of effort to push and slash through all the vegetation. But the next time you go through it is easier. As you go through the forest a lot, you start to make a path, which makes it much easier and quicker to get through – and the more so, the more it's used. It makes most sense to use this path so you do. At some point, you might go off to explore a different forest and you will have to go through the same process again there, beating out the path bit by bit. When you return to the original forest, you might find that the path is a bit overgrown. It will take more effort to get through than when the path was completely clear, but a lot less than the first time – how much easier depends on how long it's been left and how overgrown it has become.

This is equivalent to what is going on in the brain as certain connections between neurons are strengthened as you use them more. Think of all that practising times tables as slashing down brambles. The more you practise, the easier it gets. Then the summer holidays come along and you find things a bit overgrown (the neuron connections have become weaker or have even been pruned away). At some junctions, you might get confused, take the wrong pathway and make a mistake on, say, 8 x 7. But as you pick up your machete, you find there actually is a path still under there somewhere. Some connections are so strong that they never completely disappear – think of those like paving stones being laid on the path (Peters et al., 2020).

Of course, that is just one path in one forest. When you think about the fact that our brains have about 85 billion neurons, each of which has thousands of connections to other neurons, it's clear just how complicated the whole system is. It makes Ordnance Survey maps seem like a walk in the park.

SO HOW DO NEURONS ACTUALLY WORK?

Neurons are some of the most sophisticated and remarkable cells in our bodies and many books have been written just about how they function. This is not one of them! We'll instead give an overview of a few key principles.

Neurons use electrical signalling to communicate information. If you've ever seen someone looking resplendent in an EEG cap, those are measuring electrical signals coming from neurons (*lots* of neurons – one neuron on its own only produces a teeny amount of electrical energy). The power of the brain comes from its connectedness. Think of it like the internet. Any one website alone isn't going to change the world but billions of sites connected together have done a pretty good job.

The strength of connections between neurons determines the extent to which activating one is likely to affect the activation of the other. If I say 'cat' and ask you to think of a connected word, you're very likely to think of 'dog' but quite unlikely to think of 'coalmine'. The main way that the brain acquires new knowledge – or motor skills or other abilities – is by changing the strength of connections between neurons. The more connected they already are, the easier this is.

Because of the way the brain works, what we think of as 'knowledge' doesn't exist in one place; rather, it lies in the in-betweens, the connections between the neurons that hold elements of that 'knowledge'. Think of that cat again. Your understanding of a cat comes from bits of information lying in connections between neurons in the visual cortex (to picture the cat), bits of information in connections in auditory cortex (to imagine its miaow or its purr), bits in somatosensory cortex (to imagine what it feels like to stroke it), bits in language areas that tell you about the word meaning, or that said aloud it rhymes with 'hat' and 'mat'. What we think of as 'knowledge' is widely distributed.

You might see that there's a problem here. Unlike in a computer, where information can easily be moved around (just turn the information into digits, put those digits in a folder, name it, move it somewhere else), with the brain, information can't easily be moved. The transfer of memories to long-term storage involves replaying the information during sleep so that the cortex can change its connections to store it, a process that can take days or weeks.

The way memory works has other consequences. We've seen that memories are not something we put away in a mental cupboard in a fixed form; they are brought, electrically, to life every time we visit them. Their organisation is more like a website which constantly changes its links to other websites on the basis of new information. This is why it is easier to build memories on to pre-existing knowledge – the new knowledge is not a new separate entity, but a connection to that old knowledge. So if you know a lot already, adding new information is easier. Say you have the knowledge that birds lay eggs, then I tell you about a bird called a 'smew'. Even if you've never heard of a smew, if I ask you if a smew lays eggs, you'll look to your existing knowledge that birds lay eggs to find that the answer is yes. This is also how the memory trick of hooking new knowledge (say, an item on a shopping list – strawberry jam) to existing knowledge (say, a piece of furniture – a red sofa) can help us to remember it: we are co-opting the system to that end.

A final important principle is that the brain builds itself. A bit like a termite nest, where there is no master termite designer, the brain builds itself with no blueprint for its endpoint. Genes lay out some general rules, but it is chiefly a combination of chemical signals from the environment and interactions between neurons which determine the final structure. The brain is literally constructed by experience, with plenty of trial and error along the way.

Just on that, error sounds bad but actually, mistakes are catnip to the brain. When teachers encourage students to learn from their mistakes, they are singing from the brain's song sheet. Because the brain works by building up predictions about the world (as we will explore more in later chapters), it is highly sensitive to times when those predictions go wrong, i.e., when it makes mistakes. Surprise is a formidable teacher. When the brain makes a mistake of prediction, it produces a specific type of electrical error signal, its way of saying that things haven't turned out as planned. This helps to prompt a change in behaviour – typically either by improving accuracy directly, or by slowing down to improve the chance of an accurate response (Overbye et al., 2019). This same mistake system works for all kinds of mistakes, including social errors. Which is probably fortunate, if you want to avoid embarrassment.

LET'S TALK ABOUT FORGETTING

Have a look at these examples (Table 1.1).

Table 1.1 The forgettable and the unforgettable

Things I might forget	*Things I probably won't forget*
The name of someone I just met	That I'm afraid of dogs
8x7	Where I was in the first Covid-19 lockdown
The capital of Peru	How to tie my shoelaces
That dolphins are mammals	The smell of coffee
What I did on my sixth birthday	What I did earlier today
The words of a speech I'm giving	The lyrics to a song I loved in my teens

Why is this? Why does some stuff in our brains cling tenaciously (even if we don't want it to) while other stuff (sometimes stuff we really need) slips out like an eel? This seems like a design flaw. And given that learning is really all about maintaining knowledge and skills, it's also very annoying. What's going on? What is it about how the brain works that makes this happen? By the end of this book, we hope you will understand why – and it is pretty important when we think of the classroom which is all about making new knowledge and skills stick.

WHAT THIS BOOK ISN'T

This book is not going to equip you with long Latin names, wow you with kaleidoscopic images of brain scans or blow your mind with incredible statistics about the brain. It also won't be explaining much about the methods used by neuroscientists – the physics of an MRI scanner, or the electrophysiology of an EEG are not on our syllabus (with one exception in Box 1.1 'Tools of neuroscience'). There is a Resources section for those who would like to delve more into these topics and we certainly hope to have whetted your appetite. Our main goal is to give you a better understanding of two things. The first is of how the brain actually works and what its priorities are – and the implications, flowing from these priorities, for things likely to help or hamper learning. The second thing we hope to give you is an appreciation for the need for educational neuroscience; we would like you to come away convinced of the benefits of using convergent evidence from across disciplines – brain-level understanding, existing knowledge of human and social psychology, and teacher expertise – to improve outcomes for students.

WHERE ARE WE ON THE EDUCATIONAL NEUROSCIENCE JOURNEY?

These are early days for this new interdisciplinary endeavour. There is still much groundwork to be done – even at the simplest practical level of establishing networks of communication, and certainly in terms of developing pathways to the sort of evidence we want – that is to say, based on research that is rigorously tested in the lab as well as adapted for the real world of the classroom. There are some useful new resources, such as the Educational Endowment Foundation's 'Teaching Toolkit' in the UK: https://educationendowmentfoundation.org.uk/education-evidence/teaching-learning-toolkit; there's the similar What Works Clearing House in the US: https://ies.ed.gov/ncee/wwc/. While these are not strictly 'educational neuroscience' applications, they share the goal of using evidence to look at what works and why – and of freely sharing information. They also evaluate interventions in terms of how effective they are, that is, how much improvement do they bring about, and at what financial cost. Certainly a step in the right direction.

There have also been changes to teacher education in the UK. The most recent government programme 'Early Careers Framework', which outlines the training and mentoring that new teachers receive, now includes evidence-based content from the learning sciences. There is greater consideration of the role of memory in learning and of differentiation between memory systems. For example, the Framework proposes that teachers should learn that 'Long-term memory can be considered as a store of knowledge that changes as pupils learn by integrating new ideas with existing knowledge' while 'Working memory is where information that is being actively processed is held, but its capacity is limited and can be overloaded.' There are also numerous practical applications of this knowledge for teacher practice – using many of the evidence-based approaches (such as spaced learning, retrieval practice, chunking, etc.) which we endorse and will discuss in more detail in Chapter 7. These changes, again small, are nonetheless welcome.

What about the future? When people hear 'educational neuroscience' do they picture children with electromagnetic helmets siting in classrooms being 'cognitively enhanced'?

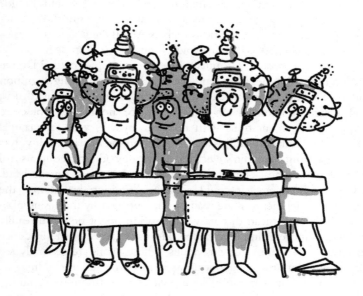

Trials are under way in China for the use of electroencephalograms (EEGs) in classrooms.[4] The headwear measures electrical signals from

4   'China's Efforts to Lead the Way in AI Start in Its Classrooms', *Wall Street Journal*, 24 October 2019 (Wang, Hong, & Tai, 2019).

neurons in the children's brains and, through an algorithm (developed by the US company BrainCo Inc.), translates these into attention scores. The children start their school day with mindfulness meditation, enhanced by 'neurofeedback' which tells them (and their teacher) how good their focus is. As they move into active learning, their teachers (and parents, who can log in remotely) get real-time data on each child's concentration. Theoretically this means that teachers can see where they might need to intervene to give help or encourage a child to stay on track. What else might it mean? China sees the artificial intelligence sector as key to its next phase of economic growth. With access to a sample of quarter of a billion or so student brains, that's a pretty impressive database.

There is much that sounds spooky, but one – some would say the *primary* – goal of the education system is to enhance children's cognition. Beyond traditional teaching methods, how far should this go? We are already using neurostimulants to help cognition: slow-acting psychostimulants treat conditions such as ADHD and are also sometimes used (illicitly) by neurotypical students to help them study. What about an everyday stimulant like a strong cup of coffee? Do we make a distinction between remediation (that is, improving cognition for those who have a particular difficulty) and enhancement (that is, improving cognition for anyone)? If we do, should we? These are complex ethical questions with no clear answers yet. Transcranial Electrical Stimulation (tES) is another tool on the horizon; it involves directly altering the brain's electrical activity by administering a small amount of electrical energy through electrodes placed on the head. Lab research suggests it could enhance cognition by altering the extent to which neurons are ready to fire, potentially increasing plasticity; this could mean that new information might be more readily integrated into existing knowledge. However, most of the evidence currently comes from studying adults, whose brains are generally less plastic; questions remain about using such approaches in children.

Genetic research is another area where new findings are raising ethical questions. The latest research in the field means it is now possible to produce a 'polygenic score for education' – a prediction generated from an individual's DNA about their educational potential. In principle, this score could be available shortly after a child is born. However, the predictive reliability of this DNA fortune teller is as yet weak, and we don't know what to do with such information. Is this even knowledge we want to have about our children? The science might still be at an early stage but now is the time to start thinking seriously about the ethical and social questions raised by these sorts of procedures.

Other technological advances hold potential for the developing field. 'Personalised learning' means learning geared to the particular needs of the individual, adapted and fine-tuned to maintain just the right level of reinforcement and challenge to maintain motivation. It is not easy for a single teacher to manage 30 individualised programmes of learning. Computer-based tutoring, underpinned by artificial intelligence and machine learning, can potentially help here, with adaptive programs, tailored to each individual user. Just as Facebook can tailor ads to swing elections, perhaps technology can tailor learning to swing exams! Again, we are not there yet, but this is an important time to consider what our educational goals are and how flexible we are in the means by which we achieve them.

More broadly, there are some tensions that continue to exist in the field about what it can and should be. Some researchers see educational neuroscience as more akin to a basic science, albeit on topics relevant to education, while others, probably most, see the translational component as key – how does this research apply to the classroom? More subtly, there can be a tension that while researchers are focused on investigating *how* something works, teachers are often more interested in *making it work*. While a researcher wants to try and isolate the exact element of an intervention that brings about change (a bit like the active ingredient in a drug), teachers are focused on improving outcomes so might prefer a broader 'throw everything at it' approach. This latter approach maximises the chance of a good outcome but makes it hard to determine precisely what brought it about. By focusing on the active ingredient, the goal of the researcher is to develop techniques which can work at scale and which can apply to a wide range of children and contexts, by showing where it is and isn't OK to be flexible. It's saying, 'You can change everything about this technique when you use it with your children, except don't change ingredient X!'

A final source of tension is in policy. Policy-makers are often interested in national or regional level policies (such as bringing in phonics screening for all 6-year-olds, a policy introduced in 2012; Standards & Testing Agency, 2011). Researchers must be clear whether such prescriptive policies are their goal – or whether they are interested in providing effective tools which teachers can then choose, using their professional expertise, whether to use, thereby supporting teacher autonomy. Cultural differences can make such discussions difficult since while debate and disagreement are the norm within scientific research, policy-makers require clarity and consensus for decision-making. Researchers need to adapt and evolve clear communication strategies.

Most neuroscience is not relevant to education, just as most education is beyond the reach of neuroscience – it being about social, political, financial and cultural questions. But there is a place of intersection, where brain-level evidence can provide a new source of knowledge about how learning works, with important application to the classroom.

Over the coming chapters, we will explore this place of common ground. We will begin by outlining some broad principles about how the brain works, based on its evolutionary origin. This means considering those aspects of the brain which rank higher on its priority list: moving and sensing, as well as meeting our emotional and social needs. We will then tackle thinking and learning, things which are really hard for the brain; there's a reason we like to sit on the sofa and veg out in front of a movie. With the groundwork done, we will circle back to the classroom and consider what all this means for teachers, using some specific examples from literacy, numeracy, the arts and the sciences. We will finally bring it all together, stressing the importance of new interdisciplinary skills which allow the best minds to bring together the best evidence in the best way, and sum up our vision for how we can bring about a quiet, considered, carefully evaluated revolution to our classrooms.

I WANNA WALK LIKE YOU...

INTRODUCTION

Evolutionarily speaking, the main reason for having a brain isn't to ponder calculus but simply to coordinate movement. In this chapter, you will meet a small part of the brain which contains a whopping 80 per cent of its neurons. You want to guess what that part does? It delivers smooth, automatic motor movements. It pours the tea, if you will. Eighty per cent of the brain's neurons! That's how important movement is. We need a way to bring together the information from our senses in order to react to it — by doing something, taking some kind of action. Even what we think of as high-level skills are based on this same process. Take attention. In the classroom context, we think of being able to pay attention as a high-level cognitive skill, but in the brain, it isn't some abstract part of thought: it is about orienting — with sight, sound, or smell — to objects in the world and getting ready to make the right movement in response. Alligators have been around for about 180 million years; their predatory behaviour involves lurking, lying perfectly still, sometimes for hours, before the right stimulus — a vibration picked up by a skin sensor — prompts them to suddenly lunge and eat whatever poor critter caused the stir. That's attention for them. And it's what our attentional systems are founded on.

Evolution doesn't reinvent, it adapts. Innovation in brain function usually involves co-opting part of the brain adapted to do something else and tweaking it to meet the new demand. A good example is our visual system, selected to be able to recognise objects and scenes in the

DOI: 10.4324/9781003185642-2

outside world, but adapted to allow us to read (when our ancestors got around to inventing the written word). The trouble is, it doesn't work perfectly for this new purpose; natural selection didn't give it the thumbs up because of its reading ability. To give an example, early visual experience leads to the development of *invariances* – if we're using our vision to drive our behaviour, we need to ignore the orientation of objects when we're identifying them. A cup is still a cup, even if it's upside-down or if we see it from the top or the side. Then we try to do reading with this beautifully developed visual system and... well, step forward the letters b, p, q, d, or the numbers 6 and 9 and we have a serious problem. It suddenly *really* matters which way round these go and whether they are upside-down. No wonder it can take years for children to learn that these special 'reading' objects play by different rules.

This chapter introduces the concept that learning in the classroom essentially rests on using our sensory and motor systems in ways for which they were not selected by evolution, ways that have been invented and honed by centuries and millennia of culture. The implications of this – from holding a pencil, to hearing rhythms in phonemes, to paying attention – are profound.

WHAT OUR BRAINS WERE BUILT FOR

Let's go back to our alligator friends. They've been around for millions of years longer than we have. And despite the fact that they have very little cortex (the outer layer of the brain that we have a lot of), they do pretty well for most behaviours (Amthor, 2016). Well, yes, you might be thinking, but alligators don't do a lot of actual *thinking* – that's obviously what humans need all that clever cortex for. Here's another surprising thing: our brains at birth are indistinguishable from those of humans born 10,000 years ago, before the first written word (Sigman et al., 2014). The same brain that used to spend its days hunting, gathering, and carving the odd stone tool can also, it turns out, enjoy the musings of Dorothy Parker. In later chapters, we will look at what has brought about this change (spoiler alert: it's to do with how super social and intensely cooperative we are, a product of our cultural rather than genetic evolution; Heyes, 2018). For now we are more interested in the things that unite us.

THE BASIC LAYOUT

To get the gist, we're going to spend a little bit of time on the organisational set-up of the sensory and motor systems of the brain. Bear with us, because it will help map out the foundations of the same systems we use for learning and will be highly relevant when we step back into the classroom.

Both motor and sensory systems are organised in hierarchical structures. They start simple at the bottom and, as information passes up through each level all the way to the top, get more complex. If you think of a skyscraper, from the lower floors, you can't see much except what is immediately outside the window, but by the time you get to the top, the view all around is much better. In the brain, the penthouse floors have a better view for two reasons: first, there's all this information being fed up to them from the lower levels and, second, they can just see more because they are higher up – they can see across to other skyscrapers as well as down and around.

How the system works is all to do with pattern recognition – finding patterns in the information that is coming in. The lowest floors spot patterns in sensory information – light or sound particles or information from sensory receptors on our skin – the next floors find the patterns within those patterns; the next floors look for patterns within the patterns within the patterns – and so on, with ever increasing complexity.

Taking an example in the visual system, light input might first be processed in terms of the general pattern of light and dark, whose features are then integrated to produce edges and curves, whose shape and patterns are integrated to produce something three-dimensional, whose movement in space produces something like a long body, the patterns of whose shape and movement produce the outcome of 'a snake'. All the while, signals flowing the other way (from the top to the bottom of the skyscraper) are feeding down expectations, based first on context (am I in Birmingham city centre or the Australian outback?) and then also on the basis of input (the accumulation of all that incoming data) of a best guess of what is being seen. If we're expecting a snake, we'll see it sooner. But too much emphasis on expectation can also mean we see things that are not there; we are expecting snakes, so we see one, whereas in fact it's only a fallen branch.

Visual illusions often exploit this idea – that our brain sees what our brain expects us to see. The visual system evolved to develop the ability to make sense of the images coming from real objects and scenes in the real world, so it tries to make sense of them within that real-world framework. That's why a 3D hole in a 2D piece of paper makes our heads hurt.

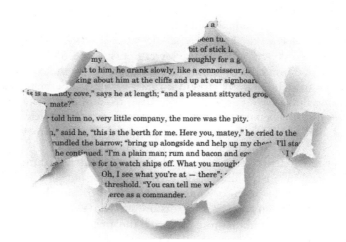

a
een tu.
bit of stick l.
my   roughly for a g
t to him, he drank slowly, like a connoisseur, l.
ing about him at the cliffs and up at our signboar.

' is is a ...ndy cove," says he at length; "and a pleasant sittyated grog
-, mate?"

- told him no, very little company, the more was the pity.

,," said he, "this is the berth for me. Here you, matey," he cried to the
rundled the barrow; "bring up alongside and help up my che-t. I'll sta'
he cont'nued. "I'm a plain man; rum and bacon and eg-   'I '
-p'   e for to watch ships off. What you mough'
            Oh, I see what you're at — there"; -
            threshold. "You can tell me wh-
            .erce as a commander.

Hole in the paper

You may have heard that the brain, or at least the wrinkly out-side layer of the cortex, can be divided into parts, or lobes. At the back of the brain, there is one lobe per sensory system: one for vision (occipital), one for audition (temporal), and one for sensing the body surface (parietal). Each lobe has a sensory hierarchy within it.

The other key ingredient is making connections *between* the top-level patterns in the hierarchies – waving across to the top of the next-door skyscraper to show off what you've got. So the top levels of the different sensory hierarchies also communicate with each other for example, to marry visual input to auditory input and agree on their interpretation of what's coming in. The sound of a 'Sssssss' helps to differentiate the real snake in the kitchen from the snake-shaped draft excluder. The top levels also connect to the frontal cortex – the planning and decision-making area sometimes described as the modulatory system, which we'll talk about a lot more in the coming chapters – to share their conclusions and see if they match expectations.

The hierarchy in the motor system has a similar set-up but the sorts of patterns here relate to their position in time. The lowest levels are based on immediate actions right now – again, think of the bottom of the skyscraper only being able to work with what is available right now, in the immediate environment. The higher you go, the more perspective you get, and the more the levels are concerned with actions further ahead in time – actions that need to be planned before they are executed. So, we go from 'Do it now' at the bottom to 'Get ready to do it' to 'Plan how to do it some time in the future' at the top.

These upper levels include complex and strategic forward planning. Imagine you want to ask someone you work with out on a date. There are lots of ways you could go about it – you could just shout out, 'Hey, you wanna go out with me?' across the office; you could saunter over pretending to be casual, 'accidentally' drop your pen on the floor and then pop the question as if spontaneously; you could send them a written message; you could persuade a colleague to put the question on your behalf. Each of these choices involves many sub-goals, each of which also has many alternative routes. (Would text or email be better? Which colleague would I trust to do this? Which pen should I drop to create a good impression of my stationery tastes?) You might run some of these scenarios in your head to try them out; running them uses the same motor circuits as you'll use once you've decided on your strategy.

Although asking someone out on a date doesn't feel like a motor function, it is only accomplished through executing a complex series of actions. The brain treats it in much the same way as it would any other complex motor action sequence – alongside and in cahoots with the emotions, which we will come to in Chapter 3.

Another important thing to know about movements is just how many are automated. By this, we're not referring to all the many movements of the autonomic system – things like our hearts beating, our lungs moving up and down, our eyelids blinking, things our brain has never had to learn how to do[1] – we mean things that we have had, at some point, to learn. Each time we get up from a chair, we don't have to think about how to do it or remind ourselves to put one foot in front of the other in order to walk over to the kettle. This only happens thanks to a huge amount of practice. Think of the hours and hours it takes babies to get good at walking – so long we have a special word, 'toddlers', to describe them in this phase. Only with practice can such actions be taken in hand and automated – writing a 'get up from chair' and a 'walking' programme and handing them over for the nerves within the spinal cord to run on autopilot.

When we're faced with a new, unpredictable situation – doing a cartwheel or tying our shoelaces – our brain has to take over and work on the problem until a 'cartwheel programme' or a 'shoelaces programme' is created. This process involves observing others, getting direct instruction and error feedback, as well as thinking and learning, that is, it requires a real brain capable of complex manipulations of the environment. It can take a very long time. But once the programmes are built, we can go back to conserving energy by running automated programmes. Such hard-won programmes are resilient. You don't forget how to ride a bike.

WHAT'S SO GOOD ABOUT *US*?

We wonder at the agility of a monkey leaping from branch to branch, or an eagle soaring then swooping in on its prey, but humans have a more complex and varied menu of movements than almost any other animal. This is partly to do with our bodies – opposable thumbs are certainly handy, standing up helps, our rib muscles allow for a smooth flow of air over our vocal cords which, coupled with our lips, tongues, and vocal cords, permit the development of intricate speech sounds. But the main reason for our impressive dexterity is our very large frontal lobes. This means we have taller skyscrapers, with many

1   This isn't strictly speaking true, since our brains and spinal cords do, at specific points of prenatal development, have to somehow start doing these things. But these functions are a product of development, rather than learned through experience and, interesting and essential though they are, they're not really relevant to the classroom. If your students are not breathing, they really shouldn't be in school.

more levels, each one adding complexity, to represent movement in our brains. The prefrontal cortex sits at the top of the motor hierarchy and it can, once developed, look the furthest forward in time – though this ability to do 'mental time travel' is not fully mastered until well into adolescence. At the highest levels, the patterns within patterns within patterns permit an impressive degree of complexity.

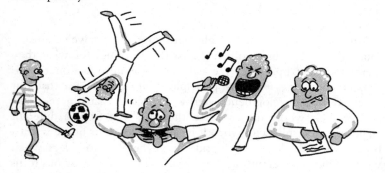

The plan for building a body with a brain goes back hundreds of millions of years. Many of the building blocks of a nervous system and brain cells – neurons, connections, electrical signalling – go back even further. Evolution tends to work from the outside in: bigger antlers, sharper claws, often things to do with the organism's movements and sensory equipment. For the brain, condemned to life inside the skull, its evolution tends to be less specific – it's not about adding in a new brain accessory for a new behaviour, it's more about modifications to the existing plan. This is why it's important to understand where our human brains have come from to give us an idea of what constitutes this existing plan.

There are some parts of the brain, such as those responsible for certain types of memory (e.g., memory of places where fear or curiosity were aroused) and arousal systems to get the body ready to fight/run/freeze/rest/eat that are relatively old[2] – our brains and the brains of chimpanzees are very similar in these areas. The cortex – the

---

2   All of the brain in your head right now is the same age. By old, here, we mean similar brain structures can be found in more distantly related species around today. These can be traced to common ancestors further back in evolutionary time.

bit that's special in mammals, enlarged in primates and biggest in humans – is much newer. In evolutionary terms, *very* new. This means that there is not a detailed, genetically determined plan for how to build all the components within it. Instead, it is almost more accurate to think of the cortex as a highly complex, general-purpose sheet of thinking power which is sculpted and shaped in response to its environment. Our brains, the most complex things in the known universe, build themselves.

Let's just take that in for a minute.

Now let's couple that thought with another one we've already touched on. The brain doesn't have to use things for what they were originally built for. We talked in the introduction to this chapter about the *invariance* principle – this is the idea that our brains, during development, learn to recognise that objects don't change their whole nature when they are seen from a different angle. A cup is still a cup when it is tipped over. Our house is still a house when we look at it upside-down between our legs when we're doing a somersault in the garden. This feels so obvious to us we can't imagine a system working another way. But then think of the child in a classroom encountering the letters b and d for the first time. Of course, they are likely to get them muddled up. They have spent literally years mastering the invariance principle and now here is something that does not obey it. It is a huge effort to unlearn it. Learning is fighting! Fighting against brain systems adapted to operate in a different world and fighting against years of learning.

These two thoughts combined – that the brain builds itself and that things built for one purpose can then be co-opted for another – demonstrate just what mind-boggling possibilities there are for what the brain can do.

We can make this abstract thought more concrete with an example from a fellow mammal. Bats are quite unusual in that they can find their way around in the dark, using a technique called echolocation. This involves the bat making sounds, then analysing the patterns in the sound waves that return to its ears to infer the location and nature of objects in its environment. The point here is that there isn't some new gizmo in the bat's brain that allows it to do this. It has evolved the ability to make the noises and it has a relatively large auditory cortex to allow for the many levels needed to see the complex patterns in the signals, but if you look at the

bat's brain, there's no 'echolocation part'. It uses the same structures as you'd see if you looked at a sheep brain or a human
brain – animals with a much greater tendency to bump into things
in the dark – but the bat has moulded them to suit its purpose.

Because some behaviours arise from repurposing parts of the
brain designed (by which we mean 'randomly arisen and naturally
selected for by evolution' – a bit long-winded and we trust you'll
forgive the shorthand) for a different purpose, they might differ
from the ideal. In other words, if we designed the system from
scratch, we might well have done it differently. Simple pocket
calculators tell us that there are much more efficient ways to navi-
gate times tables than the laborious, leaden rote learning that children have to go through. Sadly, we do not have that option. We
don't get to wipe the system and start again; we have to start from
where we are. This is a key principle. Thinking about the brain we
shouldn't be lured into thinking, 'It must be this way because this
is the best way of achieving it.' Instead, we should think, 'How
can we use our understanding of how the brain works to understand the costs and benefits of doing this particular thing in this
particular way?' What, given the way the brain works, are the
likely points of failure or the probable footholds for success? We
will be coming back to this in later chapters when we consider
thinking and learning in the classroom.

WHAT'S ALL THIS MOTOR AND SENSORY STUFF GOT TO DO WITH ACTUAL *THINKING*?

We've talked about bats and alligators, spotting snakes, learning to
do cartwheels, and even going out on dates, but this feels pretty far
from classroom learning. Surely the sort of abstract thinking we
have to do when we are working out arithmetic or pondering the
lines in a Bridget Riley painting is something quite different? Well,
yes and no.

The way that the brain abstracts (by which we mean the way it
processes information about things other than those in its
immediate environment) involves making connections between
different sensory and motor systems, under the guidance of the
modulatory system. We haven't said much about this system yet
but it's a really important one, since it's the system that is most in

control of the brain's conscious deliberate actions. We'll get into it a bit here by way of background but it will have its real moment in the spotlight in Chapter 5.

WHO'S IN CONTROL?

The modulatory system is housed in the prefrontal cortex, our bulging foreheads. Let's say it's the air traffic controller, monitoring all the flows of air traffic through the airport, talking calmly to the panicked pilot whose engine just caught fire, flitting between sets of instructions – different planes, changed flight paths, incoming weather warnings, knowing when to take a comfort break or chat to colleagues or refer something up to the boss. A lot of juggling.

There are a couple of specific things it takes care of which help us understand how it works. One is managing the 'prepotent response' (our 'kneejerk reactions') – a particular action taken in response to some sensory input that happens so often it has become automatic: putting on the brakes when we see a red light, reaching out to grab when we see a doughnut. We have hundreds of these responses, each run by an eager servant keen to spot an occasion to jump into service. But because they're automatic, they're not very nuanced; they don't know that because we are trying to lose weight we don't want to reach for that doughnut or that the red light is only for people turning right. We need the modulatory system to say 'not now, folks' and hold the servant back; it keeps behaviour tuned to planned goals, not just immediate opportunities.

A second important job of the modulatory system is to manage different sets of tasks. A 'task set' is a sort of formula involving all the sensory and motor components needed for a particular job. If I'm reading music, the C major task set means I can read all the notes straightforwardly as written, but when the piece of music changes key, the new E minor key signature task set means that now every time I see an F, I must play F#. When I'm playing 'Simon says', there is one task set for when Simon says it (that is, do whatever the action is) and another for when Simon doesn't say it (that is, do nothing). The separateness of task sets is what makes tapping your head while rubbing your tummy challenging. It's the modulatory system's job to interpret and be able to switch between different task sets.

Given its job, it will come as no surprise that the modulatory system is incredibly well connected. It could break LinkedIn. It has connections to virtually all the parts of the brain – sensory systems, motor systems, memory systems, systems for regulating the body – appetite, temperature, stress responses, hormones. It's also closely aligned with systems processing emotions and social signals and even our sense of self. It has a finger in every pie. And it needs to if it is going to pull together all the information and align arousal states, emotions and plans.

Its final key role is making decisions – even about actions stretching far into the future. If you think about it, that's quite a mental leap for a brain – to go from responding to things in the immediate environment (tasty fly, scary tiger) to planning things for the future, things which might involve many steps and detours, all carried out while keeping the eyes on the prize. Even thinking about it seems to use a lot of energy. And the whole of the pre-frontal cortex sits in a bath of neurotransmitters, which make it sensitive to how the whole system is doing – has it eaten?, has it slept?, is it stressed, tired, excited? (Arnsten, 2009). Perhaps thinking of that bath next time you fail to complete your to do list will itself be soothing.

BOX 2.1 DEVELOPMENT

Development (which is distinguished from learning by being irreversible) happens very fast early on and then slows. If we look at the brains of a 3-month-old, a 3-year-old and a 30-year-old, the 3-year-old toddler brain would be more similar to the adult's than the baby's. Just as children's bodies grow the most in the first year of life, so do their brains. In fact, babies' brains grow too much! They build huge numbers of connections between neurons, which gives them flexibility to learn and adapt – but after a while, once the brain has found its feet, they start getting trimmed away. The process is called pruning and, as with a rosebush, it allows the remaining parts to grow stronger. It is quite counterintuitive that as we get older and cleverer, our brains are reducing their connections, shrinking, getting trimmer. It's a deal with the devil: commit and optimise but lose the flexibility to adapt should the world dramatically change (at least in its sensorimotor requirements. Trip to Mars, anyone?)

With development, specialised systems get better at their jobs – more detail, better resolution, increased automaticity. Communication between neurons picks up speed as axons get coated in myelin (a bit like electrical insulation tape) which increases the velocity of electrical transmission and we see the change in the development of precision movements – that first pincer movement of a baby to pick up a small object. More effective processing also improves accuracy and means more information can be held in mind for longer (your child manages to remember their football kit *and* their water bottle). The executive (the modulatory system) takes things slower. Controlling specialised systems, activating the right ones at the right time, staying on task and planning into the future – these things all develop slowly, throughout childhood and adolescence. And working out how to operate in the world is only learnt through experience, so learning to act in a way that gets you what you want happens slowly too. By the time the brain is fully developed (typically in the early twenties), we can generally coordinate all the different parts, coalescing plans, strategies, and emotions into action.

Throughout life, spare connections are trimmed away and new connections are built. Some systems, particularly lower sensory ones, become hard to alter; this is why people sometimes talk of 'sensitive periods'. These normally refer to low levels of perception or motor output –the classic example is how hard it is to make the specific sounds of a foreign language precisely when you learn as an adult. Higher-level processing stays flexible through life. As ageing starts, reactions slow but wisdom and experience are at their heights. The healthy brain retains some plasticity for ever.

OK, let's get back to abstraction. Abstraction for the brain means having to extract overlapping similarities from specific examples – situations, actions, objects – and grouping them under a label. Let's think about the abstract concept of 'Alphabet', one of the first things children learn around the time of starting school. How the brain thinks about 'Alphabet' is as a set of situations, brought together through recognising sounds, visual patterns and making sequences of actions – real things experienced in real life. There are the letters A to Z laid out on mats in the play area; there's the alphabet song my friend sings, the muddle of letters in my Alphabetti spaghetti; there's my big sister saying 'A, B…' and pausing for me to say 'C'; there's me writing the word alphabet in my handwriting book, inside which are all the letters which make up the alphabet; there's me in my class chanting those letters in a particular order – then laughing as I try to do it backwards; there's recognising that at the start of the alphabet is A and at the end is Z. When all these real-life situations are connected and the common theme drawn from them, the child has mastered the abstract concept 'Alphabet'. The process involves the use of many different brain systems, including the key sensory and motor systems we have been describing, all brought together by the modulatory system.

We have seen that the brain is designed to recognise patterns; the way the levels in the sensory and motor skyscrapers work is by spotting increasingly complex patterns. It's something all mammals are adept at, say, for a monkey, recognising the patterns that produce the smells and sight of rotten fruit, judging the stability of a branch on an overhanging tree. This sort of learning happens naturally through experience, powered by curiosity and fine-tuned by the pains and stresses of failure.

By contrast, learning abstract concepts doesn't happen naturally. It happens as a result of being exposed to particular situations and being given direct instruction that draws attention to features that unify or separate those situations. The 'c' on that alphabet mat is the same as the 'c' you are learning to write and the 'c' sound you are hearing in phonics. Of course, language is of huge importance here in providing a shortcut to bringing together very different examples under a common label. At one level, this process of drawing attention to relevant connections and overlaps is what teaching is.

THINKING VS RUNNING ON AUTOPILOT

We have already talked about how the brain likes to automate things to ease the pressure on the system. Automation can mean developing very complex sets of knowledge about particular situations – typically those that happen often and are predictable – the sorts of things you might even describe yourself as doing 'on autopilot'. Once the brain has encountered a particular situation enough times to see its regularities, it turns the information about what usually happens into a 'script', a programme to run. If you think of brushing your teeth or getting ready to take the dog for a walk, these are complex series of actions but the scripts mean they can take place without having to think. Only when something goes wrong or is out of the ordinary in some way – a new toothbrush, the fact you can't find the dog – do we have to ease out of autopilot, adjust our attention (more on that in a minute) and begin to take things step-by-step again.

These scripts are written as a normal part of development. In fact, a lot of what babies are doing is accruing enough information from which to extract regularities to write scripts. Until that point, everything they experience is new and surprising – and a lot of work for the brain. It's one of many reasons why they sleep for so many hours each day. It's also why they like playing the same peekaboo game or singing a song many times over; repetition is a relief from never knowing what's going to happen next. A similar situation can arise in older age in people who suffer from dementia, such as Alzheimer's disease. They can no longer run their scripts because they can't retrieve them, meaning that previously familiar situations, people, and places are suddenly new and bewildering. Descriptions of perception in autism also have similarities, though here the difference is not one of script retrieval as it is in dementia but of forming predictable categories of sensory experience. If previous experience is not integrated into the prediction machinery, then there is only in-the-moment sensory input, which can make all experiences seem new and unexpected – and sometimes overwhelming.

The take-home message here is that the brain is built to spot patterns, recognise patterns it has seen before, connect patterns with other patterns, infer which patterns might appear and predict likely patterns based on context. This all happens with no need for outside input. By contrast, conceptual thinking and reasoning generally need to be taught.

MISSION IMPOSSIBLE: GETTING 30 6-YEAR-OLDS READY FOR PE

We have emphasised that the brain's priority, after keeping us alive, is its sensorimotor function, that is, processing the input coming in from all the senses and turning it into action in response. We have implied that this insight is important for later under-standing of more complex, or higher-level tasks — or to put it another way — *lower priority* tasks for the brain. Indeed, it is. How-ever, there are many things that go on in schools which do not need that extra layer of consideration, since they are themselves directly concerned with these sensorimotor functions, particularly in the early years. Here are just a few: learning how to form and write letters with a pencil and a pen (as well as underline, use a pencil sharpener, hold a ruler straight); lining up for lunch (holding a tray, putting food on it and carrying it without your water tip-ping off); getting changed ready for PE (tying the shoelaces on your trainers, putting your tracksuit on when it's all inside out); PE itself (throwing and catching a ball, doing a handstand, hitting a ball with a bat, starting to run when the whistle goes and stopping when you get to the finish line); washing and drying your hands; sitting down in your chair without making a terrible scraping sound; copy-ing a teacher's actions and performing them at the same time as singing a song; playing Champ in the playground with your friends; sitting still in assembly — the list is pretty much endless.

To carry out these functions efficiently requires a tremendous amount of practice. Some children take years to master a task like tying their shoelaces to the extent they no longer need to think about doing it until they can, literally and metaphorically, *do it with their eyes closed*. Getting these sorts of processes to become smooth and automatic involves a brain area we gave a little teaser of at the beginning; the *cerebellum* (which means 'the little brain'). The cer-ebellum is a little cauliflower-looking mini-brain found at the back of our main brain. Rather astonishingly — given its small size and lack of star power in the brain part firmament — it is so packed with neurons that it contains about 80 per cent of all the brain's neurons.

This staggering density of neurons is what it takes to keep things running smoothly. The cerebellum doesn't get much credit, because when it's working well, we don't even notice anything needs to be done. But what we think of as simple actions — lifting a leg to put on a sock — is a fantastically complicated set of com-putations involving balance, postural adjustment, sensory feedback ('Ooo, I'm toppling over'), calibration, and recalibration, all carried out by a vast number of muscles recruited to contract and relax in a dynamic, subtly adjusting, gravity-respecting orchestral manoeuvre. If you think of the pain when things go a bit wrong and you accidentally chew your cheek instead of your veggie burger or feel the weight of your body crumpling as you reach for the step that isn't there – that gives you a sense of the amazing job your cerebellum is doing, unappreciated, most of the time.

The cerebellum doesn't just do smoothness of movement, but also of thought, on the same principle of making automatic things which have been repeatedly practised. Neuroimaging studies have found that when skilled chess players are thinking about their next moves, their cerebellum is activated. What seems like abstract thought is translated into movement sequences (Sousa, 2011). When we are asking a child to practise times tables until they become automatic, we are essentially asking their cerebellum to play supernanny. As adults, if we are asked what is 3 x 3, we don't have to think before answering 9. Or what comes after 99? We know it's 100, without needing to think. Because we have had many years of practising with these sorts of numbers, we can run this sort of thing on automatic. Thirty children getting changed for PE though? That's a cerebellar minefield.

ATTENTION AS AN ILLUSTRATION

We have touched on attention a couple of times already because it is so key in the classroom. It's like the bouncer at the door: no attention, no entry to the learning party. In psychology and neuroscience, though, attention is a slightly slippery concept. A bit like 'memory', which is an overarching term for many different types of memory (and in the brain, many different systems of operation), there are also many types of attention. What holds them all together is the idea that, of the almost infinite amount of information coming in from the world that *could* be processed, our brains can only deal with a certain amount. Brains can only work well if there's some way to select which bits of information to deal with; this selection process is attention (Banich & Compton, 2018).

Psychologists use many words to describe attention. For example, *focused attention* describes the ability to maintain a focus on one thing – keeping your eyes fixed on the kettle as you pour out boiling water; *selective attention* describes the ability to home in on the thing you're interested in while blocking out distractions – reading your book on a busy train; *sustained attention* is more about the longer maintenance of attention – keeping going on a cryptic crossword for minutes or hours. Then there is the concept of *working memory* – the idea that you can only keep a certain number of things actively in mind (think of going to the shops: if the list gets beyond a few items, you probably need to write it down), which many people also describe as a type of attention (Oberauer, 2019). What are all these different attentions? How can we understand them in terms of what is happening in the brain?

Attention in the brain is the mechanism for selecting and prioritising information. The parts of the brain involved in it – the 'attention network' – are the systems (those skyscrapers again) of the senses: sight, hearing, taste, etc., and two other regions. These are a system that processes space and a motor region controlling the movement of the eyes. Let's think of our ape cousin looking at a branch swaying in the wind to decide when it's a good time to leap; attention is not some abstract part of thought, it is to do with orienting to objects in space, the thickness of the swaying branch giving information about its strength, the movement and sounds of the leaves giving information about the speed of air movement – and getting ready to make the right movement. This includes moving the eyes to look at a particular point in such a way that we get the most information from it (the centre of our eyes takes in much more information than our peripheral vision) – looking directly at the branch itself, but then to a next-door branch when the auditory system feeds in information about a loud 'crack'.

Bringing things out of the forest and into the classroom, imagine a child tidying up a room full of Lego pieces. She has been asked to sort them into boxes of different coloured bricks and is going to begin with the blue bricks. As she casts her eyes over the floor filled with pieces, she orients to and attends to pieces which are blue. This task is carried out at various places in her visual system, including a relay station called the thalamus which sits between the retina (at the back of the eye) and the visual cortex. It is responsible for *gating* – that is, changing the strength of a neuron's response to a stimulus based on the importance in a particular context of that particular stimulus. Right now, the blue Lego bricks have greater importance than the non-blue bricks, so the neurons that respond to 'blue' in the thalamus have their electrical responses *increased by the child's attention*. If she finished finding all the blue pieces and wanted to switch to finding red ones, she could switch her attention to red – and the electrical signals produced by red neurons would be enhanced instead (Amthor, 2016).

This example also points to the myth of *multitasking*, a skill which some people profess to excel at. The brain can't really multitask – because if it increases the firing of multiple neuron systems simultaneously, it's back to the problem of not knowing which to prioritise. It's a bit like at school when you highlight so many things in your book that nothing stands out any longer. The brain works by allowing competition between neurons to set the priorities for its attentional resource. Even when we think of ourselves as multitasking, what we are usually doing is, at best, a rapid switching between competing priorities, and, at worst, a bit of a dog's dinner, since every switch attempt incurs a cost as we disengage from one task and re-engage with another.

When, later, we come on to talk about *internally-directed attention* – that is, attention turned inward, to remembered episodes or concepts, rather than turned outward to things we can perceive in the immediate environment – we will see that many of these same systems are still at work. Later learning – and thinking and language – are scaffolded on these earlier sensorimotor skills, which is why helping children practise and master apparently simple activities like stacking blocks or pouring water from a jug or tying their own laces will support their subsequent development. In typically developing children, there is a strong link between meeting early motor milestones and their later cognitive development. Developmental disorders, by contrast, often first manifest first as motor problems, even if these aren't always identified at the time. It could be that these early differences alter the way in which the child perceives and interacts with the world, altering subsequent development and learning in a cascade of accumulating effects (Forrester et al., 2019; Martin et al., 2010).

In Chapter 3, we'll look at the next item on the brain's checklist of priorities: handling its emotions. The brain mostly wants a quiet life – avoiding threats, minimising stress, and trying not to think about things it doesn't like or is scared of. At the same time, it's keen to get more of the things it's fond of – friendship, bonding, feeding its curiosity. We'll see how the brain is not a battlefield where reason takes on passion (Barrett, 2018) but rather that cognition and emotion work together as an inseparable team. We'll see later that classroom learning works best when this team is flourishing as a tight-knit squad – and how dramatically it can get derailed if one part veers off track. If I am terrified of maths, things are probably not going to go well.

3

I FEEL, THEREFORE, I AM

INTRODUCTION

Our emotions are evolution's way of building basic goals – our wants – into the structure of the brain so that we can survive and thrive. Emotions are not an 'add-on', they are closely knitted to the brain's information processing systems. People sometimes talk about *cold* and *hot* cognition as if they are separate – the cool-headed calculation versus the hot-headed emotional response, but they are in fact tightly bound. There is not, on the one hand, *reason* and, on the other, *passion*; every decision we make, and every action we take, involve the emotions. And just as thinking is distributed across the brain, so are emotions.

The old-fashioned view of the brain used to be quite modular: 'this part carries out this function'. Nowadays, we realise it's more accurate to think of the *connections* between brain areas which underlie the brain's function. This evolution in our thinking is particularly relevant when we're discussing emotions, since they have historically been characterised as the 'down there' area of the brain – old, primitive, frankly, a bit embarrassing. So even when we talk (as we will!) about 'layers', it is important to recognise that there are no completely separable layers: rather, everything is connected. Emotions are more like the cheese in a cheesy quiche rather than the cheese in a cheese sandwich – interwoven, intermingled, inseparable.

With that understanding, we can talk about some degree of specialism with different layers prioritising different functions. The brain's outer cortex consists of command chains to process information relating to sensory, motor, planning and decision-making systems. Inside is

DOI: 10.4324/9781003185642-3

the older limbic system, where processing emotions and feelings are the main priority. In between lies the cingulate cortex, where all the content of the cortex above is coloured by goals and emotions below. The nature of these depends on where we are looking in the brain; cingulate cortex at the front deals with emotions around decision-making and planning, while at the back it is more concerned with how particular sights and sounds make us feel. The point is that however cold the processing of information is in the cortex; it is inextricably linked to its emotional counterpart lying just underneath.

After a brief tour of the emotional machinery of the brain, we will go on to discuss the importance of emotions in learning. Those who are curious about learning are likely to prosper, while those who are anxious may struggle. We will show why this is so, in terms of what is happening in the brain. The clear conclusion is that considering motivation, stress, anxiety and emotional engagement in learning is not an optional extra; getting these working in the right direction is fundamental to effective learning.

THE CHAUVINISM OF COGNITION

> The affective[1] side of learning is the critical interplay between how we feel, act, and think. There is no separation of mind and emotions; emotions, thinking, and learning are all linked.
>
> – Jensen, quoted in Rager, 2009, p. 25

Long before Descartes wrote his immortal words 'Cogito ergo sum' (I think, therefore, I am), the rational has always muscled into the seat at the head of the thinking table. It might be time for it to take a rest break. The more we learn about the brain, we more we see how the emotions are knitted into the fabric of how the brain works and fundamental to how it learns. Changing our perspective might mean a bit of myth busting. For instance, there is a persistent idea that lurking within our skulls is a 'lizard brain', a base, instinctual, smouldering non-human part which, thankfully, is kept in check by our all-too-human rational abilities, which prevent the desirous lizard taking

---

1   Affect is the word psychologists use for 'concerning our emotional state or our attitude'.

control. This lizard is a myth.[2] There is, in fact, only one species in the animal kingdom with a lizard brain – its name begins with an L and ends in a D. Just as our 'rational brain' has evolved over the past few million years, so has our 'emotional brain' – so that it amounts to a great deal more than a few evolutionarily ancient structures at the base of our heads. Understanding this gives us the tools to deliver better learning, since some of the greatest helpers and most forceful hinderers to learning are emotional. In fact, it is something of a paradox that some of the things which most affect learning outcomes – interest, emotional investment, engagement – are the least studied (Bell & Darlington, 2020), despite the fact, obvious to most teachers, that the way students feel can profoundly affect how they learn (Immordino-Yang & Damasio, 2007).

EMOTIONS: A QUICK TOUR OF THE BRAIN

Let's get to know some feelings-focused parts of the brain. The limbic system is made up of several evolutionarily old structures. The amygdala is best known for its fear response, working to ready the body to run or fight or freeze. It is also involved in forming memories based on fearful or anxiety-inducing situations, memories which tend to be very persistent. More recently, the amygdala has also been shown to be involved in positive emotional responses – responding to rewards and creating positive memories of events which resulted in rewards of some kind. You can think of it as the centre for appetites or preferences – storing memories of dangerous situations to avoid and attractive situations to pursue.

The hippocampus is key to making new memories. It's the part of the brain most adversely affected in Alzheimer's disease, which is why sufferers can become locked in a persistent present: they are unable to form new memories. It also plays a role in spatial navigation and orientation. A well-known study looked at the brains of London taxi drivers in an MRI scanner and compared their brains to those of other people who lacked the cabbies' refined

2   For other myth-busting around emotions as well as informative, entertaining talks and blogs, check out Lisa Feldman Barrett's website at: https://lisafeldmanbarrett.com/articles/

navigation skills (Uber drivers, maybe).[3] They found that the cabbies had more grey matter in their hippocampus – and theorised that this was thanks to the more complex navigational map they had built up over years of gaining 'the knowledge'.

As well as all their cortical connections,[4] the limbic structures are very well connected to the parts of the brain which govern the body's physical state and work to maintain our body's equilibrium. The most important part here is the hypothalamus, a tiny structure which punches above its weight, regulating temperature, blood pressure, calorie use – all the things that keep us existing in a smooth stable state. It achieves this inner tranquillity on our behalf in various ways, some through talking to the autonomic system ('Get that heart beating faster' or 'Enough with the sweating already') and others via secreting – or controlling the secretion of – a whole bunch of hormones, whose subtly changing balance profoundly affects bodily comfort.

While we're myth-busting (down, lizard brain), it is worth mentioning that, although your gym membership website might encourage you to work out to 'lower your cortisol-induced stress' or 'produce more of the happy hormone serotonin', there is no hormone that has just one single function in the brain. There are no good or bad hormones. Like so much else in life, it's a bit more complicated than that. To give an example – a teaser of something coming up when we turn to learning – a stress response in the limbic system will release cortisol which carries out a whole suite of actions in response: conditioning cortex so that working memory is reduced, impetuous responses are more likely, and learning capacity is increased. It's like the brain is focusing all its energy on responding to whatever's causing the stress and, in terms of memory, saying, 'Hey, this is really important. Make sure you remember it!' In an exam situation, this can have the unfortunate side effect that, although you could not retrieve a single piece of relevant knowledge in the exam, you can clearly and viscerally recall every precise feeling of horror and panic that came with that knowledge gap. Thanks a lot, cortisol.

---

3   See https://www.pnas.org/content/97/8/4398.full.
4   In case it isn't obvious, this just means 'connections to the cortex' – the outer layers of the brain, the tops of our skyscrapers.

EMOTIONS ARE MADE, NOT BORN

Emotions are not pre-programmed in our bodies and brains. Just like the rest of our brain, they are built. Each one of us constructs our own emotions, based on the history of our individual experiences, our bodily sensations and our environment. Even so-called 'gut feelings' are not simply visceral hunches – they are formed and continually updated through living and experiencing different situations – some with good outcomes, others with bad ones. At one extreme, they are closely tied to physiology – the disgust we feel at the idea of eating rotten meat, but even much more complex emotions – what a teenager feels when they hear a new Billie Eilish song, or the way we appreciate the creativity of an unexpected chess move, still engage the same emotional systems.

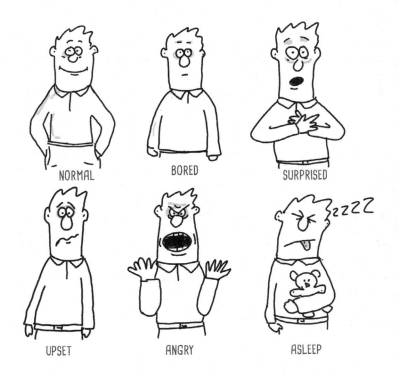

OUR EMOTIONS ARE OUR RESPONSES TO OUR PAST AS WELL AS OUR PRESENT

We can think of our emotional system in much the same way as we thought of our sensorimotor one, constantly generating predictions about the world. Our emotions are our brain's best guess of what our bodily sensations mean, based on our past experience. That sounds a bit twisty. Let's take a simple example. You have a stomach ache. Such an ache can be a sign of many different things and we can interpret this clue in different ways. If you ate some leftover chicken last night, the ache might be an upset stomach caused by gone-off food and you might feel regret that you came home late and raided the fridge. If, when you notice your stomach ache, you look at your watch and see its 2 p.m. when you usually have lunch at 1, you might well interpret the ache as a sign of hunger. If you are about to go out on a blind date, you might interpret those same physical clues as excitement. If you're about to make a speech to a group of people you really need to impress, it might be interpreted as nervousness. The same physical clue is interpreted differently on the basis of past experience and the present context. Each instance of emotion involves the whole brain, combining the past with the present, physiology with cognition. No lizards involved.

A concept that is helpful in thinking about this is that of *priors*. The literal meaning of prior is 'coming before in time or order' and in the brain it refers to all the previous experiences and learning that we bring to a situation. It is a useful way of reminding ourselves that our view of the world is always shaped by what has come before, the life we have lived. The same situation could be interpreted completely differently by two people with very different past experience. Imagine you are a child seeing a scary clown; if you have grown up in an environment where there are real scary people doing violent things, you will see that clown very differently from a child who has grown up in an environment where the only scary face they have seen is when their mum is play-acting in a game. Their priors are very different and will affect their view and experience of the world. It is easy to see how both positive and negative priors can lead to virtuous or vicious cycles, as new experiences are interpreted in old light. Anaïs Nin (1961, p. 124) expressed this idea very elegantly when she said, 'We don't see things as they are. We see them as we are.'

Another word psychologists use when they are talking about emotions is *affect*. It is closer to 'mood' or 'feeling' than emotions and can be thought of as a message from the biological organ of you. It is an account of your 'body budget', a loose sense of where you are in terms of how much sleep you've had, your energy levels, your state of hunger or thirst, whether you're tired out or full of beans. It's like a real-time, constantly updating image of our bodily state. Affect has two different axes of measurement – one is positive to negative (roughly happy/sad) and the other is high to low arousal (turned on/turned off). Everything we experience in the world is coloured by our affect. If we are feeling positive, we are more likely to interpret the actions of others in a positive way, we are more likely to give to charity, we are more likely to see the good in an ambiguous situation. If we are feeling negative, the opposite is true. It's quite useful to remember this when you are about to yell at someone after a very bad night's sleep and no breakfast.

EMOTION AND REASON

The relationship between emotion and reason inside the brain is already complex. And adding in the environment outside the brain makes things more complex still, since some situations require acting first and thinking later, while for others it is better to take time to consider options.[5] Sometimes too much rational thought is disadvantageous. A key driver for emotion in evolution was the fact that emotions allow us to *behave* in a smart way without having to *think* in a smart way. We can respond effectively to a threatening situation without having to think about it at all. This makes total sense when we imagine a deer feeling fear and running from the path of a lion. Or us not stopping to think before we dodge out of the way of an oncoming scooter.

5   Daniel Kahneman's (2012) book, *Thinking, Fast and Slow*, helped to popularise this idea of two different kinds of response: quick and more impulsive vs slow and considered.

Even in more complex human situations, behaviour that might be seen as 'impulsive' through a cognitive lens, might better be seen as 'adaptive' in the overall picture of the individual. For example, if, when you were a child, you experienced an impoverished environment where food was always scarce, then later, in adulthood, eating to excess when the opportunity presents itself (apparently an impetuous response) might be a rational response, moulded by the feeling and fear of hunger. At other times, the emotional response system might help us learn to steer clear of complex situations which might turn out to be dangerous – signalling us to pause before sending an email which our boss might take offence at. David Hume, the Scottish philosopher, strongly believed that our emotions can and should be trusted. In his *Treatise of Human Nature* he wrote, 'Reason is, and ought only to be the slave of the passions' (Hume, 1739).

Humans are capable of combining emotion and reason in a unique way, as experience and evolution have taught us to recognise the subtleties in different types of challenge from the environment. And although emotions are still sometimes seen as interfering with clear-headed thinking, when emotion is *omitted* from reasoning, reason turns out to be even more flawed.[6] The experience of communicating with a chat bot gives an idea of what dealing with an entity which can compute facts and figures but has no emotion is like. Bounded, purely logical questions can be answered capably, but any question involving subtlety, ambiguity, uncertainty, or requiring interpretation – that is, most real-life situations – cannot.

Figure 3.1 suggests a way to conceptualise the relationship between emotion and cognition. It shows that even the most high-level reasoning – such as logical thinking – is informed by emotional thought. Both higher-level areas of the brain (such as the prefrontal cortex) and lower-level areas (such as the hypothalamus and amygdala) work together to produce reason. Some

6   A famous historical neurology case was of a railway worker called Phineas Gage, who lost a large part of his brain in an accident with a crowbar. Although he recovered many cognitive abilities, the emotional component of his thinking was profoundly altered, and his friends (so the story goes) no longer recognised the thoughtful man he had previously been. See https://en.wikipedia.org/wiki/Phineas_Gage.

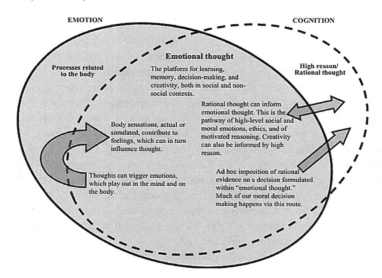

Figure 3.1 'We feel, therefore, we learn'
Source: Immordino-Yang & Damasio (2007).

describe emotions as 'steering thinking', as a rudder steers a ship (Immordino-Yang & Gotlieb, 2020). These authors describe emotional thought as something that can 'be conscious or unconscious' and as 'the means by which bodily reactions influence the mind and vice versa'.

EMOTIONS AND LEARNING

The brain networks that underlie emotional thought and keep account of our bodily state are functionally intertwined with those that underlie learning and memory. At the most basic level, if we want to maximise learning, we need our students' emotional state to align with it. When we learn, emotions are our guide to setting goals, helping us know when to push harder at a problem, or stop for a break, or try a different tack, or what to prioritise. The brain is always concerned with efficiency. A properly functioning brain will not waste energy on processing information that isn't important to the individual. To put it the other way, students will be prepared to work harder to learn skills or knowledge that they are emotionally engaged with.

This will come as no surprise to teachers. Teachers understand better than anyone how much easier it is to teach emotionally engaged students. But even though emotions are key to learning, there is a view among some educators and policy-makers that engaging the interest, enthusiasm and curiosity of students is a luxury, rather than a basic requirement. It's seen as a nice-to-have, something that makes things easier, as opposed to something without which learning – by which we mean forming, con-solidating and retrieving new knowledge rather than something woolly – will not successfully happen. This view is sometimes held particularly strongly for students who are struggling academically – those who, in fact, are often the most in need of extra help to create a strong emotional base from which to learn. The reality is that if students are pushed to learn things they are not engaged with, they simply won't remember as much. Emotion helps people attend to, assess and react to their environment – situations, stimuli and the actions of other people. Further, emotion helps the inte-gration of what they have attended to and assessed in their knowledge structures and memory, meaning that what has been attended to is remembered more. So learning is maximised when emotion is harnessed the right way.

The job of turning this into action for teachers is incredibly difficult. To begin with, if a child is not learning well, it can be ambiguous as to whether they are struggling to learn (due perhaps to some underlying learning difficulty) – the *can't* – or whether they are not motivated to learn (because they are not engaged with the material or the educational context) – the *won't*. Unravelling this ambiguity for a given child can be very time-consuming. Once it is established that the difficulty is not one of inability but moti-vation, it is still a real challenge to harness emotions in the 'right way' for learning.

There are many emotions students might have in the classroom, even positive ones, which might not help learning. If they are feeling excited about an after-school club or dwelling on hopes of getting a good score in a test, or wondering if their friends will like their performance, then the emotion can get in the way of learn-ing. In these cases, the emotion and the content of learning are not on the same train; the tracks which keep conceptual understanding and emotion moving in the same direction have split. This is one reason why external rewards – like offering money as a prize for completing homework – often don't improve learning and can even be undermining. The homework might get done, but at the expense of deep understanding and self-propelled interest. As we will see, extrinsic rewards *can* be effective – but only if they motivate the child to enter a learning situation where self-propelled interest can then take over. Another counterintuitive example comes from making school activities exciting, fun and action-packed; although this approach can improve enjoyment in the moment, it tends not to improve deeper understanding – again because emotion is not being harnessed in sync with learning. It's the difference between going on the school trip and writing the report about it.

Harnessing emotion successfully means aligning emotions with the content being engaged with. This requires the expertise of skilled teachers. A student who expresses an emotion through a story or poem in a way that authentically presents their perspective and has an emotional effect on others is likely to have a rich learning experience. A science experiment might harness the curiosity of students who want to find out what will happen and then seek to understand *why* it happened. Curiosity is a basic, motivating emotion for all mammals – mice will accept even small electric shocks if it means being able to explore a new part of their cage. Following and feeding genuine curiosity are likely to result in rich learning. As is the learning of a student who feels proud of having mastered a new concept in maths and who experiences the satisfaction of being able to transfer this knowledge to a peer. Effective educational approaches take advantage of each student's feeling that what they are seeing, hearing and learning is important, that it matters. Engaging emotion this way is sometimes thought of as a sort of gateway to learning – the way in – but it is much more fundamental than that. Engaging emotion well makes the learning itself better. If we return to our brain's list of priorities, it is not surprising that emotions can actively block learning. Negative emotions draw the brain's attention (Figure 3.2). Imagine a student in a classroom who hears an alarm going off in the building. Experience has told him that this is a sign of danger. In a worst case, it might be relevant to his survival, so requires his brain's full attention.

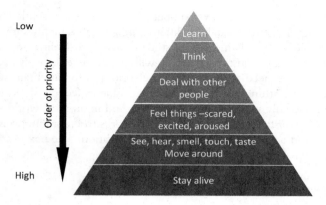

Figure 3.2 The brain puts emotions pretty high on its priority list

According to its priorities, the brain will process data affecting survival in preference to anything else. Even if the threat is perceived as lower (reduced from a survival threat to a mild fear, say) this processing will still win out over whatever the class content is.

Threats and negative emotions affect the coding of information that is key to memory processing. The prefrontal cortex is essential for retrieving and activating knowledge; when it is hijacked by the limbic system in a stress situation to organise a response to the threat, it cannot activate the knowledge it needs. This is why stress around exams can be so damaging; the stress literally makes knowledge difficult or impossible to retrieve. Even skills which are really well practised can suffer from the effects of stress. As we've seen, the brain is very good at running well-rehearsed programmes on automatic – think of the pianist who knows a piece by heart or the footballer who has taken a thousand penalty shots – but when stress enters the equation, it often brings with it self-consciousness which alerts the cognitive control system to keep an eye on performance. Disaster! Suddenly there's a back seat passenger shouting out a load of unclear instructions and everyone ends up confused and stressed. The system, fine-tuned to run smoothly and effectively on its automatic motor pathways, chokes.

The emotional contribution to learning can be conscious or unconscious. While the alarm bell is a clear example of threat, anxiety, fear and uncertainty can operate at a much more subtle level, and the level of emotion felt by different individuals is highly variable. But the consistent theme is that students who are feeling anxious, bored, stressed, or just disengaged, will not learn effectively. As a minimum, we need to align the higher priorities for the brain with the goals of learning – that is, ensure that students feel physically safe and emotionally secure in the classroom. And in an ideal world, we use our understanding of how the brain works to enlist emotions to support and enhance learning goals, i.e. motivation. The next section looks at what that might mean in practice.

MOTIVATION

Motivation is the difference between intention and action (Churches et al., 2017). *Intrinsic motivation* comes from within, when we are engaged in an activity that is aligned with our needs or desires. *Extrinsic motivation* comes from the outside, usually in the form of rewards – praise, prizes, stars, good grades. The distinction is important because, while all the evidence points to intrinsic motivation being invariably a good thing for learning, extrinsic motivation is a bit more of a mixed bag. Even apparently straightforward things, such as giving praise (a kind of social reward) can sometimes produce unintended negative consequences – for example, a student might interpret positive feedback as expectation, potentially creating stress and a sense of pressure that might reduce the success of subsequent learning.

On the other hand, carefully deployed, extrinsic motivators can help in the early stages of getting students started on a project – in a way that, hopefully, helps them find intrinsic motivation. Approaches which prompt 'situational interest' might involve actions as simple as offering choice (say, in learning materials, task, or type of assignment) or introducing a surprising new element to a lesson to heighten attention, can be successful. Underlying situational interest is the concept of 'transfer' – the idea that a positive aspect of learning in one environment can transfer over to improve learning elsewhere. We'll be talking in Chapter 7 about how transfer in learning has been something of a holy grail, as researchers have sought that magical ingredient (a skill, a mindset) that can be trained and whose benefits cascade to all learning (spoiler alert: we haven't really found one!). Here, the ingredient that is transferred is positive emotion – curiosity, interest, intrigue – the hook that is needed to get learning over what can be a tricky early stage.

Think of a class about to start studying 'The Taming of the Shrew'. One teacher starts the lesson, 'OK, we're going to try and get to grips with a new Shakespeare play today'; another puts on a video of the movie, *10 Things I Hate About You* (a modern take on the sex war comedy) and pauses it midway through a scene, leaving students on a cliff-hanger. The positive emotions stirred by the second case – interest, curiosity, attention (in contrast with the quite possible fear, anxiety or boredom invoked in the first) transfer to the next stage of the lesson, enhancing learning (Sousa, 2010).

Motivation is often considered in terms of rewards and punishments. There is little evidence regarding the effect of punishment on learning, though theory would predict it might have adverse effects, through inducing fear or anxiety – and there is some tentative evidence from adolescents (showing they are more influenced by reward than punishment; Blakemore, 2018b) that supports this. There has been more research interest in the role of rewards – usually in the form of praise – in learning. The evidence suggests that the most effective praise is authentic (that is, given when it is deserved and credible), rewards the attainment of specific pre-set goals and uses learners' own accomplishments as the basis for praise. This latest aspect links to 'growth mindset' approaches (Dweck, 2006), for which there has been great enthusiasm in the past decade. With a growth mindset, students see success, achievement and intelligence itself not as fixed or pre-ordained, but rather as the end product of work and effort. The emphasis of praise, in this view, is similarly more on the effort put in than the result achieved. The theory, that growth mindset works through harnessing intrinsic motivation, is sound, but there is a need for more rigorous research on its benefits in practice (Ng, 2018).

Recently, attention has turned to the potential for using gaming approaches to help motivation. It's hardly surprising. We watch children spend hours and hours playing video games and wonder what it is that makes these games so compelling. They seem to produce the ultimate intrinsic motivation environment. We know that the hormone dopamine is associated with responses to reward – and that increased dopamine is associated with a faster rate of learning. More specifically, dopamine release is affected by whether a reward is expected or unexpected or of uncertain nature (think Wheel of Fortune). The *anticipation* of a reward (whether the reward is something fundamental to well-being, like food, or something more subtle, like verbal praise) is sufficient to initiate a dopamine response – and the response is increased if there is a degree of uncertainty about whether the reward will be realised (Howard-Jones, 2015).

This idea, which emerged from a scientific look at how games so successfully hook attention, formed the basis for a classroom intervention where, instead of getting set points for a correct answer, children got a range of rewards determined by the spin of a fortune wheel.[7] The trial highlights some of the difficulties of putting educational neuroscience theories into practice. The results did not show the expected effect (that is, children in the unpredictable reward group did not learn better than the control group) but the real difficulty is that the significance of this finding is hard to interpret, since only a minority of participating teachers actually carried out the intervention according to the guidelines, due to logistical constraints of the quiz and game. It seems that the experiment was just not sufficiently well adapted to their classroom needs. The example also shows the challenge of linking learning in neuroscience (which encompasses multiple mechanisms) to learning in the classroom (which is measured by a change in skill or behaviour). The dopamine theory only really applies to fact learning involving the hippocampus – so even if it were successful, it might not extend to conceptual learning and deeper understanding.

As we will discuss more in later chapters, in educational neuroscience, good scientific theory alone is not enough. Putting theory into practice means many stages, both to fully explore its potential application and to create meaningful collaborations between teachers and researchers, to ensure that interventions are planned, tested and carried out in the context of the real-life constraints of the classroom.

STRESS

All animals are adapted to handle a certain amount of stress. It's a necessary part of being able to adjust to uncertainty in the environment, for example, by maximising the ability to fight or flee from a perilous

7 See https://educationendowmentfoundation.org.uk/projects-and-evaluation/projects/engaging-the-brains-reward-system.

situation. The typical stress response involves increased heart rate and blood pressure, decreased salivation and digestion, sweating and a relaxation of the bladder and rectum. This is quite a dramatic impact on the body, all in order to optimise the body to act right here and right now.

The response to stress is highly individual – the same amount of outside stress will affect each individual differently. To further complicate matters, not all stress is bad – the evidence suggests there is an optimal level of stress for learning – a level which brings about an alert engagement somewhere between sleepy/bored and anxious/overwhelmed. Stress also varies by the type of task; it can increase attention and learning in some situations but hinder it in others, as shown in Figure 3.3.Figure 3.3(a) shows how arousal levels (an approximation of stress) and performance are related: poor performance is associated both with not enough and with too much arousal. Figure 3.3(b) captures an extra layer of subtlety – that the relationship depends on the nature of the task. For difficult tasks, the same association holds, but simple tasks seem more resilient to even high levels of arousal.

There is another important distinction, which is between short- and long-term stress. Short-term stress – or acute stress – is a response to an immediate, finite situation (a hidden person jumping out and shouting 'Boo!'). Long-term stress – or chronic stress – comes from things which have no clear start or end (perpetual loud noise outside the window, a chaotic environment with a lack of time for relaxation or no personal space, more serious examples, such as parental abuse or

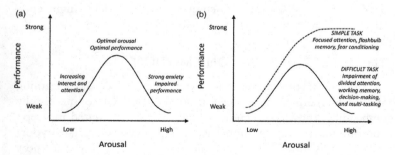

Figure 3.3 Relation between arousal levels and performance
Source: Whiting et al. (2021).

neglect). These chronic stressors have persistent effects on body and mind – they tire the body and exhaust the mind almost as excessive exercise does. Children who suffer from chronic stress experience the world differently; for example, children who have grown up in an environment of psychological or physical abuse are likely to be more vigilant and to have difficulty focusing attention. On the other hand, children growing up in chaotic environments are sometimes particularly skilled at problem-solving in challenging contexts, since that has been their training ground and they have had to learn to cope (Evans & Kim, 2013). There's also some evidence to suggest that differences in learning outcomes arise depending on whether stress is perceived as a debilitating factor or an enhancing one; is a challenge something to be afraid of or something to embrace (Immordino-Yang & Gotlieb, 2020)?

The timing of stress is yet another complicating factor. If a moderate amount of stress is part of a task – the stress happens along with the task – it can enhance learning. But stress that comes before or after a task can have a negative effect. This is because stress directs the memories that are formed most strongly; memories relevant to the stress are prioritised over those which are not. So if learning comes before or after stress, the learning itself slips down the priority list and its content can get lost.

Stress encompasses a complex set of responses which are still a poorly understood aspect of learning. The hope is that future research will help clarify the circumstances which will best enable learning for different pupils. For now, it remains an enormous challenge for the classroom, since the environment which might produce the best learning outcomes for one student might constitute too much or too little stress for another.

THE EFFECT OF SLEEP ON EMOTION

We will be talking more about sleep when we consider learning and remembering, since sleep is so fundamental to successfully embedding knowledge. Here, though, we are interested in sleep's contribution to our emotional state. If you've ever dragged yourself grumpily from bed to frowningly face the day, you'll know what we're talking about. There are two aspects we are interested in: one concerns our natural circadian rhythms, the daily fluctuations of hormones which govern our basic functions – breathing, temperature, digestion; the second is the sleep cycle itself.

The timing of our circadian rhythm is driven by our exposure to daylight. There is a natural daily cycle, that means we are on peak awareness between about 7 a.m. and noon, then a lower level of awareness which declines from about 2 or 3 p.m. onwards. There is a trough that occurs in the early afternoon – typically between 12 and 2 p.m. for pre-adolescents and about an hour or two later for adolescents. This is a time when learning – and teaching, since teachers also experience this slump – are much harder work. Early afternoon is not the time to be tackling the hard stuff.

A good deal of recent research has explored the change that takes place in this daily cycle around the time of adolescence, with an emerging picture that challenges a still-prevalent view of adolescents as lazy slugabeds. In fact, the changes in hormones around the time of puberty have a huge effect on their circadian cycles, shifting them later: they get tired later in the evening, and they stay tired later in the morning. On average, adolescents don't reach a time where their brains are primed to learn until about 1–2 hours later than younger children. For this reason, there has been a great deal of interest in studies to look at whether changing school start times might improve outcomes for this age group – though the logistical hurdles are enormous. A more moderate response to these scientific insights is to tailor what is taught at different times of the school day. For adolescents, this might mean using the first period for tasks which are educationally valuable but make low demands on the prefrontal cortex, which is particularly affected by low arousal states.

The second issue concerns the quantity and quality of sleep itself. Sleep has a pivotal role in determining how we build our emotional world. It is crucial for all healthy mental functioning – a lack of it particularly impacts the modulatory system, so that concentration cannot be sustained for as long, mental flexibility is reduced, and impulsivity increases. Insufficient good sleep interferes with emotional regulation, increasing irritability, frustration and anger and with social functioning, makes us less tolerant of others and more likely to be inflexible and dogmatic. This combination of an amplified response of the amygdala (making it more likely to interpret emotional stimuli

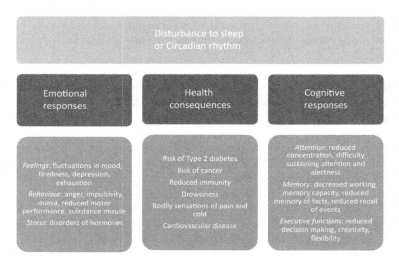

Figure 3.4 The many consequences of sleep disturbances
Source: Based on Sharman et al. (2020).

as negative or threatening) and the reduced communication with the prefrontal cortex (which would normally keep an eye on this sort of drama and calm things down) are what can make those who haven't had sufficient sleep so edgy to be around.

Figure 3.4 highlights the many effects of disturbance to sleep and circadian rhythms. The consequences of sleep disruption cover a broad range from relatively mild effects such as frustration and tiredness caused by short-term sleep problems, to serious health consequences of long-term disruption. Those on the left of Figure 3.4 concerning emotional responses are the ones we have discussed here. We will come to the cognitive responses, which are concerned with learning-relevant processes, in later chapters. But the point again is to think in terms of the brain's priorities; if our emotions are not up for it to begin with, learning will be an uphill battle.

TEACHERS HAVE EMOTIONS TOO

Before we leave this chapter, we wanted to give a quick shout-out to teachers. Although our focus in this chapter has been on the brains of students, everything we have said applies equally to those whose job it is to teach them. If teachers are tired, stressed and unmotivated, this will have as profound an effect on their ability to teach as the same features have on their students' ability to learn. In fact, you could argue that it will have 25–30 times the effect, since teacher performance will impact each and every student in their class. Keeping teachers healthy, well-supported, well-nourished, well-motivated and unstressed isn't just good work practice, it's good science.

In Chapter 4, we will tackle the next item on our brain's priority list. It's also one of the most complex things our emotional systems have to deal with. Other people.

NO ONE IS AN ISLAND

INTRODUCTION

A great deal of what occupies the brain is other people. We are social primates, meaning a lot of our brains end up being concerned with processing social information. It also means we are very affected by relationships – with families, with friends, even with strangers – and by figuring out where we are in any hierarchy. Among social primates, the larger the social group, the larger the cortex – suggesting that processing all that social information takes a lot of brain power.

There are many ways our brains are specialised for processing social cues. Our visual systems are more tuned to movement that comes from people than things, our auditory system has special pathways for distinguishing human speech from other sounds, and our limbic systems help to generate the myriad emotions linked to social actions. More complex systems allow us to verbalise our thoughts and emotions to communicate with others.

As we grow up, just as we learn the links between different bodily feelings and action (I recognise I am thirsty so I drink a glass of water), we start to learn social conventions (when I see someone I know, I smile and say hello). As we become more adept, we make connections between ourselves and what we observe in others; we see someone else crying and not only do we recognise that they feel sad, but we feel sad too. But the loops from limbic emotion systems to the outer cortex mean that even empathy is always dependent on the specific context: we only feel sad if we like the person. We cry for lifelong friends experiencing adversity

DOI: 10.4324/9781003185642-4

but sworn enemies (players from a rival football team, say) can crash and burn!

This chapter considers the importance of other people in effective learning, with clear implications for the nature and importance of the teacher–student relationship, as well as for the role that our peers play in our learning.

SOCIAL REALITY

If you think about the world, there are many physical realities: the tree growing in the park, the river running through it, the fox that raided our rubbish bin, atoms which make up matter, the shrinking of the Dead Sea. All are physical realities. Then think of another set of things: the borders of countries, a person in charge of the country called a Prime Minister, exams that can be passed or failed, money that is exchanged. These are not physical facts but social facts. They are things that have come to exist in the world because at some point humans decided they were a good idea. The world we operate in on a daily basis is mostly this invented place rather than the physical one: we go to school, or to a place called work and write words in documents or cast votes in ballots for elections which make some people move out of a house and other people move in. All these activities follow complex rules, built up sometimes over centuries; we must learn how to operate within these rules, learn what is and isn't acceptable, what will or won't get us socially censured. Much of this is stuff we are never taught but are nonetheless expected to understand – and go along with.[1]

Creating this complex social reality is what makes humans unique as a species. How we have come to acquire this ability is still something of a mystery, but most scientists agree it requires a combination of skills that are much more developed in the human brain, at least by adulthood. Some call these special thinking tools

1   Of course, some of the most exciting moments in history come when people decide not to go along with it, but rather to change the current version of social reality. Decisions not to go along with social norms underlie big changes like the Civil Rights movement or women's emancipation and smaller things like fashion choices or whether it's OK to look down at your mobile instead of up at pedestrians while walking on the pavement.

our *cognitive gadgets*.[2] They arise from using some ordinary, evolutionarily bequeathed cognitive tools in new and flexible ways, that is, they arise more as a result of using the same things differently, than having different things to begin with. Another way of thinking of this is that they are the product of cultural rather than genetic inheritance, passed on through people rather than through DNA. We develop better brains thanks to social interaction.

There are some particular specific skills that have allowed us to develop this complex world. Our creativity allows us to come up with things that did not previously exist – to use our imaginations to see possibilities that are not there in our environment. Our communication skills allow us to pass new ideas on to others. Communication is also a fantastic shorthand. A simple statement, such as 'I'm standing for school council' conveys a vast amount of information – imagine how much you would have to explain if you were saying this to someone who didn't know what each of those words represented – how complicated it would be, how many words it would take. But with interpretation also come many assumptions which can lead people down wrong paths, often without knowing.[3] As well as creating and communicating new ideas, we need people to be able to replicate the ideas and cooperate to put them into action in other places. Think of money. Money works because it is an idea that many people buy into, and which persists because many people cooperate with and reproduce the idea, to the extent that it becomes a social reality. If you ask someone to explain money, they will probably offer some idea that money works because of some kind of guarantee by a nation state – that's why the Queen has her picture on our money. Even though that guarantee is just referring to another social reality – since we could all decide one day that our nation state, or the royal family, should be got rid of – it seems more concrete than a piece of paper. Concrete enough that we go along with it. Then along

---

2   Celia Heyes (2018), *Cognitive Gadgets: The Cultural Evolution of Thinking* is a great book on the subject.

3   People with autism sometimes have difficulty understanding idiomatic expressions ('You are driving me nuts', 'That's the last straw') since understanding these expressions depends on figurative rather than literal interpretation.

come cryptocurrencies, virtual money in video games and non-fungible tokens, and slightly blow our minds.

We don't give much thought to these sorts of things. But looked at afresh, it is unsurprising that it takes a lot of brain energy to learn, carry out and automate all these complex social programmes.

THE HEART OF THE MATTER

Emotions are an essential component of understanding and negotiating social exchanges. These exchanges are the some of the most complex situations humans have to deal with. That's why soap operas, or books by Jane Austen, or dramas about the mafia, or reality shows about people falling in love (or pretending to for the money) or ... well, an awful lot of culture, is given over to poring over social interactions. It's probably the thing we as a species are most gripped by. And across animal species, the most intelligent animals tend also to be highly social.[4]

Understanding people and understanding emotions are inextricably linked. Emotions are the legal tender in the world of social interaction, since other people have such a profound influence on what is going on in our own brains and bodies. You smile at me; you change my hormone secretions! You say something horrible and bullying, my brain predicts threat and issues urgent supplies of other hormones. Other people can be the best things for our brains and bodily health. People in loving relationships – whether with family members, partners, friends or even pets – are ill less often than those who are alone – and are even more likely to fight off serious illness. It's actually pretty incredible to think that a hug emoji received in a text from a loved one the other side of the world can change the hormone levels in my body!

But the converse is also true. The flip side of our dependence on other people is that others can also have profoundly negative effects on our brains and bodies. People who live in violent relationships – and who experience regular physical verbal or emotional abuse – not only suffer the acute effects of these aggressions (the immediate stress response), but also the effects of chronic stress. These can include

---

4   Those dastardly octopuses, as with so many things, generally buck this trend.

anxiety, depression, increased risk of heart attack, sleep problems, digestive problems, headaches and impairment of memory and concentration. There is almost no bodily system that is not adversely affected by persistent abuse. Less extreme situations can still have dramatic impacts. In overcrowded urban environments, where large numbers of people live close together, the stress of living constantly cheek by jowl with others raises the underlying risk of mental illnesses, such as schizophrenia, through adversely affecting the 'social stress' network in the brain. The neuroscience implicates the anterior cingulate cortex (which is involved in regulation of amygdala activity, negative affect and stress) for those brought up in urban environments, and increased amygdala activity for those living there right now and not enjoying it (Lederbogen et al., 2011). City living shows how the social and the emotional are tightly linked for the brain.

THE WHAT'S WHAT OF WHO'S WHO

When people talk about the 'social brain', they are not referring to a particular brain area responsible for the social stuff. There are in fact many different systems in the brain with a role in processing information about other people. Given that social interactions include activities as diverse as catching a glimpse of a sudden human movement out of the corner of your eye, to hugging your grandma, to responding to a prosecutor's questions in a court of law, it is clear that managing all of this will draw on many brain systems working together in a coordinated way. Basic sensory systems are specifically tuned to human sights and sounds; other systems allow us to infer what is in other people's minds; the mirror system helps us understand what other people are trying to do – by actually replaying the same actions in our own brains; all these operations are set in the context of the social world, with its learnt rules and behaviours. Some systems operate involuntarily – being able to differentiate human movement from other types of movement, for example[5] – while others are deliberate – using our expressions to convey additional information to others; a raised eyebrow is sometimes enough to tell you 'I don't believe a single word of what you just said.'

---

5   Such is the brain's power to spot human movement that you can detect characteristic actions, such as a figure walking, when it is represented by no more than a few moving dots of light.

When we talk about social cognition, we mean two things: learning *about* other people and learning *from* other people (Frith & Frith, 2010). Let's get into a bit more detail on the systems which control both of these.

LEARNING ABOUT OTHER PEOPLE

From the moment they are born, babies start learning about other people – what do they look like? Smell like? Sound like? Feel like? What effect do they have on me? Evolution has rewarded us for being able to recognise other people – as collaborators or competitors, kith or kin, potential mate, or potential adversary. From birth, our brains are tuned in to differentiate the signs of people from all the other stimuli in our environment and prompted to learn more about them.

OUR SENSES ARE TUNED TO THE SIGHTS AND SOUNDS OF HUMANS

Most mothers cradle their babies on their left side (Forrester et al., 2019). This is true even if the mothers are left-handed, so doesn't seem to be to do with keeping the dominant hand free for other activities. Rather, it seems to be an intriguing clue about the earliest social processing that happens between babies and their carers. How does it work? There are a few things to know: first, the right side of the brain (and left visual field) tend to be particularly attuned to social processing. Second, the left side of our face (controlled by the right side of the brain) tends to give stronger emotional signals than the right side of our face.[6] So cradling on the left does two things: it means the baby's emotions are signalled most effectively to the mother (giving access to her left visual field and right side of her brain) and it means the baby gets easier access to the more expressive *left* side of its mother's face. This in turn allows greater bonding and social development. The point here is not that cradling is a hugely important factor by itself, such that bonding might fail without it – in fact, the difference between left and right cradling on social development is tiny. We use it here as an illustration of how it is a combination of hundreds, thousands, tens of thousands of tiny activities which together shape development. There are very few

6   See Blackburn and Schirillo (2012).

absolute 'rights' and 'wrongs' of good development and a large number of 'Well, this might be a little bit better'. Reassuring for parents and carers and a big 'to do' list for researchers.

The visual system has pathways that, over the course of development, become increasingly specialised to recognise human faces.[7] These same pathways also recognise and differentiate between facial expressions and make interpretations about the particular emotions they likely convey. The subtleties of what expressions represent emotionally vary somewhat between cultures. Although people typically recognise all emotions with a fair degree of accuracy, they are more accurate when it comes to recognising expressions by members of the same national, ethnic, or regional group as themselves. The more contact they've had with people outside their own group, the more accurate they are likely to be, since the greater level of exposure has meant their brain has had the chance to learn the finest grain distinctions between faces (Elfenbein & Ambady, 2002). The brain learns about faces, as it learns about everything: through experience.

The visual system is also geared to recognise the specific movements of people, that is, to differentiate human movement from the movement of other animals or things. Even very young infants can distinguish human from non-human movement. Many different types of sensory information – where the person's body is, how it is moving, what shape it is – are brought together to allow us to recognise people from all sides, when their back is turned to us, when they are running or standing or sitting, or when they are outside of their usual context.[8] We are skilled at understanding the movements involved in gestures people use to communicate. And just as the visual system is tuned in to human movement and expression, the auditory system is specially adjusted to attend to and process the sounds of human speech, as distinct from the many other sounds in the environment. If you imagine picking out the sounds of what your friend is saying even when the rattle of the

7   Some people have great trouble recognising faces; the condition is called prosopagnosia. You can find out more about it at: https://www.troublewithfaces.org/.

8   Though seeing people outside of their usual context (e.g. a child seeing their teacher in the local shop) presents additional processing challenges.

Tube train makes the words barely audible, that's thanks to how socially attuned your auditory system is.

MAKING SENSE OF MOVEMENTS

Even when we are looking at objects which don't seem to be human, we attribute meanings to actions. Figure 4.1 is part of a simple animation involving two-dimensional shapes moving around on a screen. It was developed to analyse the tendency to attribute meaning nearly 80 years ago.[9] Shown the animation, most people do not describe the movements in terms of spatial dynamics and the trajectories of different shapes (e.g., both triangles move upwards at a 45-degree angle), but instead use terms which give human-like motives to the inanimate shapes, for example, here one triangle (or 'resident' of the 'house') might be seen either as 'inviting into' or 'expelling' another triangle (or 'friend' or 'family member' or 'enemy') from entering the

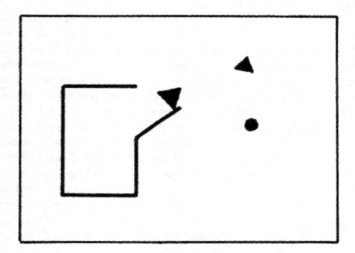

Figure 4.1 The social brain can make even simple geometric shapes into complex human stories
Source: Heider & Simmel (1944).

9 See Heider and Simmel (1944).

'house'. We naturally attempt to infer meaning from movement, based on our understanding of how humans operate in
the world. It can sometimes take great effort *not* to anthro-
pomorphise, since doing so is really the by-product of our social
cognition.[10]

When we see another person moving, we want to interpret that
movement: what is the person doing? What is their goal? Again,
even very young babies do this. The understanding that human
movement, unlike a flower wafting in the wind, is not random,
but carries a meaning of a person's underlying goal, starts young.
And in the same way as we do with our own bodies, we try to
predict the movements of others. We do better if we have some
knowledge of who they are, what they have done before and what
they might be thinking. We can get clues about whether another
human might be like us. For example, people copy each other. It's
usually unconscious, but when we connect with someone, we tend
to copy their movements and their gestures – scratching our chins
when they scratch theirs.

Mirror neurons, first discovered in macaque monkeys, are neurons that fire both when an animal performs a specific action and
when the animal observes the same action performed by someone
else. The importance of mirror neurons has sometimes been exag-
gerated, for example, calling them our 'empathy cells' since they
literally recreate in one person the feelings and actions of another
person. In reality, although these neurons seem to have special
capabilities, they are essentially operating as most neurons do when
they are completing the (admittedly quite miraculous seeming)
activities of action prediction. We saw in Chapter 2 that the sensorimotor system works both in terms of sensory-up input and
brain-down prediction, using the same circuits for both. Mirror
neurons are better thought of in the same way. The same neurons
that enable you to give a 'thumbs up' to tell your friend they did a
good job also help you interpret someone sticking their thumb up

10 Perhaps you can spot a link here. We saw in Chapter 2 that the visual
system's years of experience learning to recognise objects whatever their
orientation then makes it hard for that visual system to learn written letters. Similarly, years of the brain learning the dynamics of social movements then make it hard to see shapes following those same give-and-
take trajectories in a non-social way.

to you as meaning that they think you have done well. These emulations of actions are so strong that professional tennis players can improve their play simply by practising their moves in their heads (Frank et al., 2014).

Babies are masters of the imitative arts. But when they are using their mirror neuron system to imitate others, is it to mentally re-run a movement in order to work out its goal, or is it the internal activation of a goal that has already been worked out by the brain's prediction machinery? An intriguing study on 1-year-old babies tried to find out (De Klerk et al., 2015) by looking at what happened in the babies' brains as they watched an adult trying to kick a ball. Would they copy the action of leg movement, or the goal of moving the ball from A to B? Well intriguingly, their brains showed activation in the area representing their arms rather than their legs. One-year-olds generally cannot kick, so if they wanted to move a ball, their best bet would be to use their arms. This suggests that their copying is even more sophisticated than a simple facsimile – they are copying the *intention* rather than the *mechanism* of the action programme.

MIND READING

We use our experience of who usually does what, who they do it to, how other people react, how all this makes us feel, where we are in the pecking order – to build up ever more complex programmes about social behaviour. We build predictions about what other people are likely to be feeling and, using our own emotional experiences, what they might do next. This process is called mentalising and is like a kind of mind reading – all still based on our best guesses. We see someone else reach for the biscuit tin; we might think, 'They're hungry' but we might also add experience and context and instead think, 'They're feeling sad', or 'They're trying to steal the chocolate ones before their little brother gets home.'

Another step involves actually empathising with other people's feelings. We recognise certain behaviours – sad faces, slumped shoulders, heavy walking – as meaning that someone else is feeling depressed. And we feel sad too. We often mimic their sad face and their slumped shoulders and their heavy walk. Even if we are just watching a movie and we see someone getting hurt, we respond physically and emotionally – we flinch as they are about to get hit. As ever, we are combining sensory input coming in with predictions coming down. Our frontal lobes remind us that the guy about to get hit is the villain and our empathy level plummets.

When we communicate with other people, we make assumptions about their mental states, based on our own. Even here, and as with the motor system, the brain likes to run things on autopilot as much as it can. We saw in Chapter 3 how we build our emotions by learning to make links between certain feelings in our body and needs that we have in the world. We link a feeling of hunger to the desire to eat and the action of going to the biscuit tin (and past it to the fruit bowl if our modulatory system is having a good day). In much the same way, we learn about other people through starting to recognise signals from the outside world. Just as we run motor programmes, we learn to run social programmes. This is a combination of the work of the frontal cortex to combine its own goals with context and emotional states in order to tell motor and sensory systems to behave in an appropriate way. I'm walking into my classroom in the morning so I must calmly say 'Hello' to my teacher before I sit down quietly at my desk. Now it's break time so I can run around like a crazed banshee shouting and flailing about with my friends. Different social programmes.

LEARNING FROM OTHER PEOPLE

Picture the toddler putting on rubber gloves and washing up their doll's tiny tea cups in the sink or holding a phone and yelling into it just like Mum does or digging in the flower bed just like Dad does. Imitation is an efficient way of learning.

OTHER PEOPLE HELP TO BUILD OUR BRAIN

Social learning can be efficient because we can learn from watching other people get things wrong and correct themselves, instead of having to go through each learning journey ourselves. Social learning is also a kind of double learning – we learn about the person as well as the content. If we see someone spell a word wrong, and then, being told of their error, we see them laugh off their mistake and give it another go, we are learning something important about dealing with setbacks as well as how to spell. Our brains are well adapted to learn from others, because we use the outcomes of *their* learning as another way of updating our 'priors' – that sense of what the likely outcomes are. Other people are a great extra source of information to make our own decision-making better. As with all learning, social learning updates the information in our brain by changing the strength of connections between neurons. Social learning is the brain's constant attempt to minimise the disparity between what it thinks will happen and what actually happens. When we get something wrong – that is, our predictions were off – we are surprised; our brain is particularly attuned to this surprise and makes sure that we learn from it.

Different types of people tend to be important as our teachers at different ages and stages of development. In the early years, our primary carers are our main source of learning. Our brains are built to learn from them, by the attention we pay them and the reward we feel by gaining new knowledge – and their brains are rewarded by helping us. When we get to puberty, this shifts and our peers often become a more important source of learning. Teachers, of course, are unique, in that they are the only people whose job it is to daily alter the brain connections of their students – and they must do it over a whole age range. In the next short sections, we will consider these different groups in a bit more detail.

LEARNING FROM PARENTS AND CARERS

Social skills are visible at a very young age, even from birth. Newborns show a preference for human faces and human voices over other stimuli. They follow the gaze of other people to get more information and they react to other people's communication attempts (Frith & Frith, 2010). Although we can learn a great deal just by watching other people – and many animals do this – deliberate teaching seems to be, even among primates, particularly human. Studies on very young infants (around the age of 6 months) show that when carers give simple signs such as saying the baby's name or making eye contact with them, infants are more likely to follow their gaze afterwards than if no such clue is given. The cue serves to help orient infants towards that element, in an environment filled with stimuli, which is most likely to give them rich information. The communication of information is inculcated as an expected social act from infancy onwards (Senju & Csibra, 2008).

When infants start learning words, this orienting ability is critical. As we have discussed before, many of the 'new' things that our brains do (by 'new' we mean on an evolutionary timescale, so things like reading) are achieved by borrowing functions of the brain that came about for other purposes and co-opting them for the new one. Chief among the language-relevant abilities is the ability to infer the intentions of others (Bloom, 2002). Infants can distinguish, for instance, between a situation in which a parent is specifically naming an object for them to learn and one in which an object and its spoken name come together by chance. This learning is only made possible by the social nature of the communication (Baldwin et al., 1996). Even more impressively, toddlers can use their mentalising ability (that is, their ability to put themselves in the mind of someone else) to tell the difference between someone who knows something and someone who doesn't – and to pay more attention to the one with the knowledge. So infants and young children are highly skilled both at selecting the most reliable signals and prioritising those with the intention of communicating – all of which helps them to learn words at the astonishing rate they do.[11]

LEARNING FROM PEERS

During adolescence, the teenage brain undergoes big changes in its mode of operation and in its pace of learning, especially for certain abilities and domains. This has only come to be appreciated in the last couple of decades (before then, it was assumed that most brain development was done by the start of secondary school). Some even refer to this time as a 'sensitive period' for sociocultural processing (Blakemore, 2018b). The changes in operation are

---

11   Ten new words a day, according to Bloom (2002).

triggered by alterations in motivations and rewards, linked to the hormonal changes of puberty. They make for a discontinuity in the environments teenagers put themselves in and the experiences that they learn from: they don't want to hang out with boring parents any more, they want to hang out with their cool friends (and they really want to impress them). Two brain systems are particularly affected. First, the prefrontal cortex, which is the buck-stops area for complex and abstract thought, future planning and the control of attention and behaviour – it's home to the mod-ulatory system we have discussed. It is still shaping into its adult form and has yet to undergo the myelination which will make it fast and efficient. Second, and under the influence of puberty hormones, are structures of the limbic system, which, as we saw in Chapter 3, is the bedrock of the emotional system.[12] The changes underpin the archetypal changes in behaviour of teens: the need for more social interaction with their peers, increased desire for sensation-seeking and the sort of risk-taking behaviour that alarms their parents.

Many of the changes are based on preparing adolescents for an independent life outside the family. A key feature is prioritising peers in information-gathering and decision-making, in preference to parents and teachers. Since part of the task of an adolescent is to develop the social skills that will allow them to prosper in adult-hood, their attention needs to be particularly focused on social interactions, just as the infant's attention was oriented to sensory systems and learning to coordinate movement.

Adolescents are highly sensitive to social rewards. This means both that they gain more (relative to adults) from positive feedback from peers and that they suffer more from negative peer reactions (Tomova et al., 2021). Hence the need to avoid embarrassment at all costs – they literally feel it more than adults. One of the key hormonal changes in puberty (in addition, of course, to changes in the sex hormones, testosterone and oestrogen) is in the levels of dopamine, a hormone we met before when we talked about reward-based learning. Dopamine is involved in activities like sensation-seeking, novelty-seeking and risk- taking – all activities

12 This combination of changes is what some describe as the 'high horsepower, poor steering' of the teenage brain.

which tend to peak in the adolescent years. But why? What purpose does this serve?

Recently, scientists studying teenage brain activity have found that when teenagers are monitored while they're playing a driving game, they take more risks if they are in the presence of peers (Gardner & Steinberg, 2005). Brain imaging shows that they have greater activity levels in parts of the brain related to reward when their peers are watching. Risk-taking in front of peers is hormonally more rewarding for adolescents than it is for adults. Simply put, such behaviours give more pleasure. This can lead to some complicated calculations for teens, for instance, is it more adaptive and a better choice to risk the health damage of smoking a cigarette than (given the importance of positive peer feedback), the possible social opprobrium of not smoking?[13]

It also offers up learning opportunities. An important aspect of learning any new skill is responding to feedback,[14] that is, how it uses information about whether we are right or wrong, doing well or badly. Feedback is related to activity in the striatum, part of the brain very involved in rewards, reinforcement learning and seeking out pleasures (even addictively). How well people learn from feedback is related to activity in the striatum – and teenage brains typically have more active striata than children or adults (Peters & Crone, 2017). This suggests that teenagers might learn better from feedback, particularly from their peers, and points to a possible role for collaborative group learning at this age.

Learning can also be exploratory – trying a sport or hobby for the first time, for example. Here too, the teenage brain responds in a special way, driven by the rewards of exploration being felt more strongly.

13 Teenagers are sometimes described as having poor decision-making around risk-taking. It might be more accurate to say their decision-making is fine, it's that they have a poor appreciation of the risk themselves. When a teenager takes a crazy risk (dancing along the top of a high wall, while knocking back a beer), it is because they think it is worth the risk (say, for the social attention they will receive). They do not yet have a balanced appreciation of risk that comes with the experience of adulthood (otherwise known as wisdom!).

14 The term feedback here refers to an internal message that the brain uses to adapt its behaviour, rather than the grades that teachers hand out.

This makes adolescence a particularly fruitful time for exploration – of self, of others, of the world. But increased sensitivity to reward can also bring negative consequences when the feeling of reward comes from drugs or other potentially addictive substances. Heightened emotional sensitivity also means that exposure to stress and social isolation can have profound long-term consequences for teens.

The overall message here is that rather than negate the social need of adolescents to learn and get approval from their fellow adolescents, harness it! If they are given opportunities for group work and collaboration which allows them to work with peers, this social motivation can provide a very powerful engagement tool. By the same token, teachers need to be vigilant when that same peer pressure is having an amplified negative effect on some students' learning.

LEARNING FROM TEACHERS

Our brains are inherently social organs. As highly social animals, we generally prefer to experience and learn new things in the company of others. That way, we can share ideas, learn from others' mistakes and benefit from the positive emotions evoked by collective success (Tokuhama-Espinosa, 2010). But in school, we also need to learn from teachers. What can teachers do, in terms of socio-emotional best practice, to ensure that things go well?

The first thing is simply to understand the importance of the social and emotional experience of each individual learner. It is not an add-on. Emotions and social needs cannot be left at the door of the classroom. They are baked in, prioritised in the very structure of the brain. As such, teachers will see the best results if they understand and work with them, not against them.

Making mistakes and getting neural feedback signals from them are key features of learning for the brain. They provide vital signals to a brain optimised to learn from when its predictions are wrong. Many studies have found that, after we have made a mistake, we slow down – this is the simplest, catch-all response to buy more processing time to avoid making the same mistake again. Our brain's response to error can be measured by changes in its electrical activity, called its Error Related Negativity or ERN, and measuring this, researchers have found that the greater the ERN following an error, the more a subsequent response is slowed down. Even more enticingly, it seems that strong ERNs are *a good thing;* in one study, students who had a stronger ERN response also had better grades.[15] Surprise is a great teacher. Learning is about being curious, exploring, testing and pushing things to see if they react in the way you're expecting – and learning when they don't. Outlawing error is outlawing one of the most helpful learning devices students have.

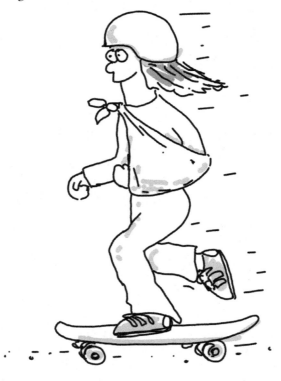

The attitudes of both teachers and students to mistakes can have a big influence on outcomes. Students are very aware of, and sensitive to, how particular teachers respond to errors and have a clear

15   See Hirsh and Inzlicht (2010).

sense of good and bad ways of responding (Tulis, 2013). To create an environment adapted to learn from mistakes, teacher responses might include offering a hint to guide a student to another response, opening up a wrongly answered question to the whole class to discuss, waiting for long enough (at least 5 seconds) before jumping in, emphasising the learning potential of an error, and standing in the way of negative reactions from other students. On the contrary, ignoring or criticising a mistake, passing the wrongly answered question straight on to another student to answer, laughing or showing disappointment or disbelief are all counter-productive. Although we have talked about the particular sensitivities of teenagers to feedback, these good and bad practices are true for students of all ages.

THE SOCIAL CLASSROOM

The good news is that optimising classrooms and teaching for social learning is no different from accepted best practice. The best classrooms are safe, calm and purposeful. Teachers help students establish a sense of ownership of their work and to feel that their work has value and relevance. They engage students with open questions, ideally related to their individual interests and experience. They identify opportunities for collaboration between students and focus them on a shared goal. They use both intangible rewards (such as praising pieces of work or particular contributions) and tangible rewards (such as house points) with sensitivity to potential unintended effects. They support both exploration and new discovery, alongside deeper elaboration for depth, and help students negotiate movement between these different approaches. They appreciate that the most effective way to motivate students is to harness, by whatever means they can, their intrinsic motivation and pursuit of goals which are meaningful to them – something that is not always easy when the more arbitrary goals of compulsory, statutory exam performance measures tend to hold sway.

There is another aspect to social learning, which applies very broadly across ages and subjects: *making content more social makes it more engaging*. And bringing a dry story to life almost always involves adding a social dimension – who made a discovery? How did they feel about it? How did other people react? What were the consequences? Who is enthusiastic to learn about Darwin, whose career depended on voyaging the world by sea, but was tormented by seasickness? Who is not keen to learn about Ada Lovelace, knowing that, as well as putting her mathematical brilliance to use on the Analytic Engine, she was also a compulsive gambler? Case studies can bring any subject to life and, if used well, can encourage students to see the world through the perspectives of other people, even those they profoundly disagree with. Personification can also be used to bring a social dimension to learning even in the absence of real-life human protagonists: the cells of the immune system recast as the cast of *Glee*, elements of the periodic table re-envisioned as characters from *The Simpsons*.

Human narratives have a privileged cognitive status (Graesser & Ottati, 1995), they are catnip for the brain. Bringing the social dimension to learning is another example of aligning the brain's higher priorities with the conceptual learning that teachers are after.

LEARNING TO BE A SOCIAL BEING

Just as the brain is built by interactions with our environment, the social brain is built through interactions with our social environment. Brain development and functioning are socially and culturally bounded – products of the sociocultural environment, as perceived and experienced by the individual. As we saw when we looked at emotions, different bodily sensations will be interpreted differently depending on the context in which they occur: someone with a pounding heart might be angry or excited or nervous, which it is depends on the context.

Over time, our interpretations of social situations feed into our sense of cultural identity. Our experiences start to reveal patterns which are more to do with groups we belong to ('woman', 'Black British', 'bisexual', 'meat eater', 'Conservative', 'youth', 'prisoner', etc.) than simply our individual identity. This adds an extra layer of complexity to the interpretation of emotional clues – now that pounding heart might signal anger caused by not having been heard on account of being a member of a particular social group, or excitement at being recognised and accepted by a group we want to belong to. Interpretations are subject to continuous cycling and updating: the interpretations I make of these social situations in turn influence what I believe, the values and morals I have, the person I become, who then interprets social situations… and so on for ever.

This system works in a very similar way to that of the somato-sensory system we described in Chapter 2. We saw that our experience of the world is determined by two things: first, by the input − processing signals from the senses, which are passed up through levels of increasing complexity to the top of the hierarchy (remember those skyscrapers). Second, by predictions coming down from the top floors − predictions based on previous experiences and current context. In the same way, our embodied brain, using its social processing know-how to operate within the cultural world, both *constructs* feelings in that context, and has emotional responses *induced* by that context, in a dynamic, constantly updating cycle.

We can crystallise this idea with an example. Let's think about a girl going in to take a physics exam. Her body is showing signs of physiological arousal which she interprets as nervousness about the test. She knows that the physics exam is important because she wants to study engineering at university and needs to do well, but she has heard her teacher make comments that suggest he doesn't think girls are good at physics. The meaning she makes of the situation leads her body to produce more stress hormones, making her heart pound and her mouth dry up. Sensing this, she feels a sense of impending doom, a sense that she is likely to fail in the exam and prove that the teacher's prejudice was correct. The ruminating uses up precious cognitive resources which actually make it less likely that she will do well in the exam.

A parallel girl about to take her physics exam starts with the same symptoms. Her teacher is confident she will do well and has told her that if she feels nervous she must 'harness the power of the butterflies'. Her parents have reminded her that, previously, when she's taken exams, she's always felt nervous but has ended up doing well. All this pours into a feeling of positivity about the challenge − and she interprets the same bodily symptoms not as nervousness but as a sign of excitement and challenge about the test − a chance to prove herself. This means she tries really hard in the exam, and her preparedness to take on a challenge helps her to retrieve memories of all those equations.

BELONGING

Belonging, that is, the feeling of being included, accepted and valued in a social group, is one of our fundamental needs (Schwartz et al., 2016). Our sense of whether we belong can powerfully affect our learning, positively or negatively: while a strong sense of belonging can boost engagement and motivation, the sense that we are not welcome, judged or subject to stereotypes (on account of race or gender, for example) can significantly increase anxiety and lead to poorer learning outcomes. Belonging is where themes of the social brain and the emotional brain come together. We socially construct our ideas about group membership: we identify in a certain way; we identify others in certain ways and this determines whether we identify with a particular group or feel we don't belong. Many students who have earned their right (through exam success) to go to university just as others have, might still feel a kind of imposter syndrome, a sense that they do not belong there. Certain actions by others can obviously increase this sense, for example, by adding to stereotype threat through conveying a sense of lower expectation of good performance on account of certain gender, racial or other characteristics. More subtly, someone's sense of not belonging often goes unidentified and unacknowledged by teachers and peers who have never questioned their own sense of belonging, meaning the student does not receive the support they need.

Interventions to improve a sense of belonging can improve learning (Aguilar et al., 2014; Walton & Cohen, 2011) by improving students' persistence even when learning is challenging, increasing the effort they are prepared to make and by their ruminating less on ideas of whether they belong. Interventions might involve efforts to change the environment, or to change people's attributions about belonging by helping them to re-envision their beliefs. For example, a student who feels she does not belong might use evidence of a disappointing exam result to 'prove' her belief that she does not deserve or should not be at college. Showing her testimonies from older college students who describe having had similar setbacks before going on to graduate successfully can help her reframe her experience as typical rather than unique to her. We know that the brain takes on new knowledge based on previous experience, so it is important to remember that outcomes – exam results, reactions even to 'constructive' feedback – will be taken differently depending on what the student has heard before, directly or indirectly.

Belonging is at the limits of where neuroscience can usefully contribute to improving learning, but some early work in this area suggests some of the specific brain systems which are important (Kieckhaefer et al., 2021). For now, the important message is to be conscious of the potent role that belonging can play in psychological well-being as well as in learning. 'The feeling that one belongs is wonderful. The feeling that one does not is awful' (Schwartz et al., 2016, p. 19).

BOX 4.1   THE NATURE/NURTURE DEBATE

At some point, we have probably all wondered how we might be different if we'd been born to different parents or raised in another setting. Would I still even be me? Teachers have more experience than most of the huge differences that exist between children, even siblings; it's natural to wonder where these differences come from. This often leads on to the so-called 'nature/nurture debate' – the question, put simply, of the extent to which we are born or made.

Let's start with some basic facts. We have fewer than 25,000 genes which somehow give rise to all the complexity of the human mind and our behaviour. The nematode worm has nearly 20,000! Simple maths makes it very unlikely, despite dramatic headlines ('a gene for obesity' or 'the gay gene'), that any gene is fully responsible for any complex behaviour. Instead, many genes interact with each other and with the environment to influence every trait. Each gene also contributes to many different behaviours. In terms of the environment – the nurture part – this includes a mind-boggling array of *everything in the world that isn't our genes*: whether our mothers had post-natal depression, what we ate for breakfast this morning, the level of our climate anxiety, whether our society is democratic, a bitter argument we had with our brother when we were 10. Just as genes interact and entangle, environmental effects interact and entangle. And the more we learn about epigenetics (that is, the study of how the gene-to-environment information flow is not one-way; that the environment also has a say in how genes are turned on and off, up and down), the less it makes sense to think of nature and nurture as separable. Genes on their own do nothing. Only by undergoing a complex sequence of biological processes, all of which are environmentally influenced, do they produce even a protein, let alone an ability to do maths.

So why are we even talking about this? One reason is that, even though separating nature and nurture itself is not particularly useful, we are still really keen to know what influences educational outcomes and how, with a view to improving them. We know, for example, that the effects of the home and family on education are bigger than school effects by about a factor of 3, suggesting it is important for educators and policy-makers to think about the wider social context for students. With more digging, we might be able to be more specific about how effects from the home and family cause particular outcomes. The other reason it's important is in preparation for the future; polygenic risk scores (which add up the many individually-tiny-but-powerful-in-combination effects of many gene variations) to predict aspects of a student's likely educational attainment are already here. There are individuals and corporations keen to use them, though they are currently a blunt instrument. Imagine an equivalent poly-environmental risk score (child was born prematurely, lives in a polluted urban environment, experiences financial hardship, has high school absences, etc. ...); equally, this wouldn't help us know whether or how to teach them differently.

In the future, genetic information might help create the best, tailored environments for individual students, targeted to their unique strengths and weaknesses. For now, we are in the soup. Our key message, for both genes and environment, is to pivot the question from *whether* they influence educational outcomes to *how* they do so. Our mantra throughout this book is to focus on mechanisms of change – how does it work?, what follows from what?, what can we influence? – because only by understanding how things work, be they genetic effects or environmental ones, can we ever hope to make them work better.

Are you frustrated? We didn't really answer the question, did we? Are differences in human behaviour more due to nature or to nurture? And how would you answer this question anyhow? One way is with twin studies. Twins, whether identical or non-identical, are typically raised together in the same environment. Identical twins are very genetically similar (same DNA, 100 per cent similar!), whereas non-identical twins are no more genetically similar on average than siblings (50 per cent similar DNA variations, on average). This means that if, when raised in similar environments, identical twins come out more similar than non-identical twins, say, in their maths ability, this is probably due to their greater genetic similarity, that is, due to nature. If pairs of identical and non-identical twins are equally similar to each other, it's probably due to the shared environments they are raised in (e.g., they have a great maths teacher), i.e., to nurture. This is one way to have a stab at comparing the variability due to nature with that due to nurture ... if you wanted to, even though we've said they're inseparable. A paper (Polderman et al., 2015) summarised the findings of all the twin studies ever carried out up to that point – a century's worth of studies involving some 14 million twin pairs. And so ... is it more nature or more nurture? The answer they found was that, for educational achievement (and most other behaviours), it was about half and half. Maybe you could have guessed that.

We have now completed our tour of the brain's top priorities: sensing and moving, dealing with emotions and understanding other people. We hope that it is clear now why some neuroscientists have suggested that 'the brain is not for thinking'; there are many other things it's simply more bothered about. Nonetheless, it does, reluctantly, do thinking. And it is to that thorny task, with thinking cap on, that we'll now turn.

THINKING IS HARD

INTRODUCTION

The brain is primarily designed to process sensory information about the world and produce a motor response. It is good at that – just think of a gibbon judging which branch to leap onto or a chimpanzee selecting out the rotten fruit. What it is less good at – and can only do with a great deal of effort and practice – is *abstracting*, that is, forming general concepts. As we've seen, the brain processes information within specific motor and sensory systems. These are well adapted to find patterns in the world and bring information together to make sense of the world and act in it. Abstraction is a whole different ball game. It requires the modulatory system to work with sensory and motor systems to pull together different information under some sort of abstract label, a process that's highly dependent on language.

Think of the concept 'six'. Understanding what 'six' comprises is quite a task for the brain. It requires exposure to many different situations, tied together by language, to understand that the six you count on your fingers is the same as the number 6 you recognise and can write. And that is the same six as the one that comes after five and before seven on a number line, or the one that you need if you're putting things into groups of six, or dividing a pizza into six parts, or producing the result of multiplying two by three, or being told how many wives Henry VIII had. When all of these diverse situations can be connected conceptually, we have mastered an abstract idea of 'six'. Astonishing really, that most children have accomplished this by the time they start school.

DOI: 10.4324/9781003185642-5

To think, we need to have input both from the immediate sensory environment and from memory. If it weren't for memory, we would have to start again from scratch with each new piece of input. Memory is a complex beast. We will be dealing with it piece by piece in this chapter and the coming ones.

This chapter puts thinking into the context of something that's low down the brain's priority list. It's further down than coordinating movement and sensory input, reacting to emotional signals and managing the complexities of dealing with other people. More fundamental priorities must be aligned for the pathways to higher-level thought to be clear. And because the brain relies on systems built to deal with specific types of content, perhaps the greatest challenge it faces – and where it needs the most support – is applying its abstractions to new situations.

WHAT IS THINKING?

It's easier to describe what thinking is than to neatly define it. It includes a diverse set of activities, including using words, developing concepts, problem-solving and mental time travel to anticipate future events or recall past ones. We can talk about logical thought, imaginative thought, emotional thought, intuition, rationality. We might add creativity, memory, communication, collaboration and learning to our list. We can go a step further to add metacognition – the very human job of thinking about our own thinking.

Perhaps the simplest type of thinking involves referring to an entry in our long-term memory, for example, the thinking involved when we try to think of an Amy Winehouse song, or a country that borders Latvia. What if we are dealing with a more complex question? Imagine being asked, 'Did the Covid-19 pandemic mirror the Black Death in how it exacerbated social and health inequalities?' You would have to carry out a complex series of mental operations, first, turning to memory to see what you have stored about each pandemic, searching that knowledge for effects relevant to inequality – after making decisions about how to define inequality – then contrasting lists drawn up for each pandemic to analyse them, comparing and contrasting. An open-ended question might demand a different kind of thinking again: if I ask you, 'What's your most unusual idea for how to drop an egg from 50 metres without it breaking?', memory will only take you so far. Instead you will have to extract rules – the conditions required to protect the egg shell from a sudden force, generate strategies and search around in a more unknown problem space that lives outside the proverbial box.

Most models of thinking comprise the sorts of stages shown in Figure 5.1. Anything seem familiar here? Remember those sensory and motor towers – start with basic-level sensory input, then analyse patterns within them, then patterns within patterns? Well, thinking is based on much the same set of processes. An important additional element concerns the allocation of attentional resource – deciding where to focus. We'll come to that shortly. The key idea here is that the brain loves to find patterns, loves to find links between different patterns, and loves to try to predict which patterns are likely to come up. It's also fine with then correcting itself when a pattern doesn't obey its predicted rules. Abstract thought, reasoning, conceptual thinking are, by contrast, not straightforward 'natural' activities for the brain. It needs a lot of repetition, strategies to follow,

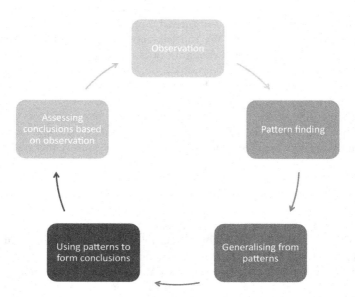

Figure 5.1 The stages involved in the thinking process

cues to prompt use of these strategies and external guidance to help it do those things. That's where teaching comes in.

THE BRAIN IS NOT LIKE A DIGITAL COMPUTER

In our quest to make the brain understandable, we often liken it to other things — it's 'like a sponge', it 'works like a muscle'. Through history, people have tended to liken the brain to the fashionable technology *du jour*: a steam engine, a telephone switchboard or, for the last half century or so, the digital computer.

This is pretty misleading. Computers work by putting all the knowledge into a common format (digits) and using a really good calculator to process it. A computer is unmoved by whether it is processing images or numbers or mouse movements or swipes of the screen. It processes them all in the same way. This common format also means that the knowledge in a computer is easy to move around — the hard drive stores it, the working memory (RAM) unit holds it temporarily and it's all fed into and out of the central processor to do the calculations, without needing to change its form. So computers are dependent on, first, the abstraction of knowledge and, second, fast movement of that knowledge between general purpose processors.

These two key processes are both things that the brain *does not do*. That's not to say it might not be better if it did — in fact, in the future, we might create artificial intelligence systems that take into account all our biological weaknesses and work better than our own brains[1] — but evolution can't start from scratch; it can only ever work with what it has. And evolution did not give our brains the tools to work like a digital computer.

Thinking of how the brain is *not* like a computer helps us understand some of the particular difficulties it has. First, how do brains do abstraction when information is processed within specialised systems (visual cortex for visual information, auditory cortex for auditory information, and so on)? And, second, how can information be moved around when the information itself lies in the strength of connections between neurons? These are

[1]   If you want to learn more about this, Nick Bostrom's (2015) book, *Superintelligence* is a good, if mind-bending, place to start.

thorny problems that are clues as to why abstract thinking is a tough challenge for the brain. Grab your swimming trunks and let's dive in.

ABSTRACTION DON'T COME EASY

The brain is a natural pattern seeker. It looks out for familiar patterns so that it can make predictions about what will happen next. It automatically seeks out patterns in new sensory experience. The systems for doing this, as we saw in Chapter 2, are built on concrete experience of the real world: sights, sounds, smells, movements. Abstraction requires the brain to step outside of this concrete world, where senses dominate and patterns are found without thinking, to a world where finding new patterns has to be taught – concepts which are either not obvious in sensory input or which involve bringing together disparate sensorimotor associations, as we saw with the number six. Because it is not what the brain does naturally, it takes a lot of time and practice.

Seeing abstraction in this way shows thinking sitting atop our motor, sensory, emotional and social bedrocks. Picture the child learning to count by touching each of their fingers in turn – this is motor movement underlying abstract thinking. For the brain, abstraction is not about separating itself from these processes, but rather aligning them in an organised way so it can pull out higher-level patterns. Let's take a trickier example: analogies require high-level abstract reasoning in order to detect the correspondence between two different things. Watch what your brain does as you try to work out which of the following pairs are analogous:

<water: pipe> and <blood: blood vessel>
<cow: milk> and <duck: water>
<tiredness: yawn> and <fear: shriek>
<basil: herb> and <oak: tree>
<puppy: dog> and <cat: lion>

To do this, you use all the lower-level sensorimotor systems to visualise each item (or even enact them bodily – did you yawn when you read 'tiredness: yawn' or grimace as you read the word 'shriek'?) and keep the relationships in mind while the modulatory system directs attention to particular mappings to test their correspondence. Your brain takes the lower levels and adds attention to find the mappings which produce an answer. (Answers: Yes, no, yes, yes, no. How did you do?)

Although it is hard work to begin with, if we have sufficient practice, we can start to run mental simulations on automatic.[2] That's what philosophers do when they pull out logical arguments on demand, as the rest of us would instinctively put out a hand to catch a moving ball.

MOVING KNOWLEDGE AROUND

What about moving knowledge so that it can be found again in the future? And does it even need to be moved? To answer this, we must distinguish between different types of knowledge, since they are handled differently in the brain. The key distinction is between conceptual knowledge (the type we have discussed under 'abstraction' above) and what is called 'episodic' knowledge (the type that concerns particular instances). Instances are specific autobiographical moments – how I wore my hair yesterday, my friend's text saying he has a crush on Tom Holland, what I am eating right now. But, of course, these two types of knowledge do not remain completely separate: knowledge networks are built up out of multiple instances. The instances of knowledge which fill a classroom lesson – this fact about this country, this new piece of vocabulary, the lyrics of this song, this historical date, this moment my friend explained it – have to make their way into knowledge networks – to be connected to other knowledge, to enrich understanding, to be applied elsewhere, to aid future learning. The instances *feed* the knowledge networks, so they create a situation where knowledge *must* be moved around.

Another key point (one we will be returning to and elaborating in coming sections) is this: instances can be learned fast – it happens

2   For example, for our analogies, figuring out that you should articulate the feature that relates the first two words and check if it also relates the second pair, and then automatically applying this strategy.

in the hippocampus (part of the limbic system),[3] which can change its connections very quickly to record instances as sort of snapshots or video clips. By contrast, learning the associations between knowledge and fitting them into conceptual structures is slow; it is handled by the cortex, where changing connections between neurons takes hours and is mostly done while we sleep. So building networks of knowledge cannot be done fast – both because of the time taken to gather the experiences of different instances – life! – and because of the time taken to weave all those instances into ever-shape-shifting knowledge networks.

So how does it actually happen? How does that new fact you have just learned about Black Widow become integrated into your extensive knowledge of the Marvel universe? We know that knowledge exists in the connections between neurons in different regions of the brain, so this seems like a tricky problem. It's so tricky that to do it, the brain has to be taken off-line during sleep. Even then, it takes hours to move information around – an incredibly laborious process compared to the microseconds it takes a computer. During sleep, the hippocampus takes centre stage; as we've said, it is the key actor in transferring information from short- to long-term memory – in neuroscience parlance, taking the information that has been *encoded* (that is, processed by the senses) and *consolidating* it (storing it). More accurately, it is the connections between the hippocampus and the cortex which are key. Here are some important things to know about that system:

- While we are asleep, the hippocampus spontaneously replays the events of the day – the information that has come in from the senses. When that information comes in, the hippocampus creates a kind of 'snapshot' memory, combining all the sensory input.
- There is a key 'loop' between the hippocampus and the cortex. By a loop, we mean neural connections. The connections from the cortex to the hippocampus cause synapses relating to particular memories in the hippocampus to be

3   Remember the limbic system is a key emotional hub for the brain. The fact that the crucial area for forming memories is located in the midst of that emotional heartland is significant, as we will see in more detail later.

strengthened. These strengthened synapses, in turn, connect back to the cortex.

- This means that key parts of the cortex (those which correspond to particular experiences) can be activated from the hippocampus rather than from sensory input.
- The cortex can recreate a version of the same neural activity that took place when the experiences actually happened.
- Long-term memory resides in the same parts of the cortex as were involved in the original experience (when you remember something vividly, you can almost re-smell or re-see or re-hear the sensory experience – because the same pathways are being activated).
- Almost *the entire cortex* connects to the hippocampus and back again. This is not a small backroom operation; this is Glastonbury Festival.
- The process of memory consolidation can take several days and even weeks to complete.
- The hippocampus eventually fills up. A rough estimate is that each hippocampus (there's one on each side of the brain) can hold about 50,000 memories of specific situations or experiences.
- This is all quite mind-blowing! Most neuroscientists were surprised to find that memories exist in the same place as they were first encoded – so if this is news to you, you are not alone. How it works precisely is still the subject of much active research.

We will be going into more detail about memory shortly, so this is just a starter – to demonstrate how memory in the brain and memory in a computer are very different beasts.

GUIDED BY EXPECTATION

Another important difference between brains and computers is *prediction*. The brain does not just sit and wait for things to happen. It is constantly building predictions about what will happen next, based on what has happened before. That's why you might trip up if someone has put an unexpected object in a familiar setting, or why a child might shrink from his mother's dramatic new haircut. We saw in the earlier chapters that the brain develops *scripts*, blueprints of how things usually go. Scripts take a while to build because they need multiple occurrences of the same or similar experiences. When it comes to new things, there is no script. For babies, everything is new. That's why repetition (routines, songs, games) is so soothing – it is a relief to be able to run on autopilot. Scripts run for social and emotional events as well. If we go to the party of a new acquaintance, we draw on our knowledge of what parties are usually like in order to predict how this one will be and how we should act. We know how we will feel if we watch a horror movie because we've seen scary movies before. We know the rules.

There are two reasons this is important. The first (touched on in Chapter 4) is that when predictions are *wrong*, it is a powerful prompt to thinking. We talked about the fact that mistakes present opportunities that can potentially be exploited in the classroom. The second is that prediction is a balancing act. If you *over*-predict, you miss things – it's called 'inattentional blindness' – you don't see something simply because you did not predict that it would be there.[4] On the other hand, if you *under*-predict – that is, you fail to take prior experience into account and are constantly being driven by present sensory input – the world is constantly new, with everything unexpected. That can easily get overwhelming. This is how people with autism sometimes describe their experience of perception.

So let's sum up where we are so far on the tricky job of thinking. We have said quite a bit about how the brain is not like a digital computer and the consequences of this for abstraction and moving knowledge around. We've also shown how heavily the brain relies on prediction. We'll now take things on to look at how what you learn depends on what you already know, and this is a stepping-stone to understanding the importance of memory. We're going to have to do a bit of work there, to find out what different memory systems there are (bear with us!), and we'll also find out about the importance of forgetting. We will finally give our first shout-out to the very human and quite sophisticated skill of thinking about

4   Have a look at this to get the idea: https://www.youtube.com/watch?v= vJG698U2Mvo or if that's too easy, try this one: https://www.youtube. com/watch?v=ubNF9QNEQLA.

thinking. This will set us up for the crucial topic of Chapter 6 (for teachers, at least) – how the brain learns.

EXISTING KNOWLEDGE MAKES NEW KNOWLEDGE EASIER TO LEARN

The American Psychological Association defines knowledge as 'the state of being familiar with something or aware of its existence, usually resulting from experience or study'.[5] The definition captures the idea that knowledge comes both from direct sensory experience *and* from making sense of experiences. Knowledge can be unconscious (I know how to walk but I don't think about it) or conscious (I know that I can tell you the first three lines of elements in the periodic table). It can be easily accessible (my name), slightly harder to access (what I wore to work yesterday) or really hard to access (capital of Malawi). Some knowledge I have stays with me forever (what my sister looks like), some might drift away (the recipe for brownies).

There's another complication. Much of what we learn at school does not come from direct sensory experience but from *report* – what other people have found out. This raises other issues, for example, social questions (Do we trust who the report was from? Should we? How do we feel about authority figures?) and also the challenge that the easiest way for the brain to learn reported knowledge is through the sensorimotor learning required to reproduce it – that is, rote learning. Most teachers probably recognise the effort involved for students to put something 'in their own words' or in not just repeating something back 'parrot fashion'. There's a reason parrots do it that way! The challenge then is to go the longer route to build the knowledge networks that can regenerate the reported knowledge.

How do you induce conceptual understanding from verbal reports of knowledge? It's not easy. The learner must extract the sensorimotor basis of the intended knowledge with models, diagrams, mental images and relevant actions, all of which are no more than indirect indicators of the target knowledge. Let's say a teacher wants to explain how to measure the event horizon of a

5   See https://dictionary.apa.org/.

black hole. This is tricky for students to experience directly in the average classroom, without imperilling all of life on Earth. To induce this conceptual knowledge indirectly involves gluing together concrete models (black hole = something physical and spherical) with abstract concepts (mass, gravity, spacetime, singularity) via language; and practising the motor plans and procedures that should be linked with this conceptual knowledge (drawing a picture of curved spacetime, writing out and manipulating the equations for the effect of gravity on light). The challenge of indirectly inducing conceptual knowledge through direct sensorimotor experience and language instruction in the classroom is to ensure that the correct aspects of these experiences are incorporated into the concept, and not irrelevant information from the experiences used to transfer the knowledge, such as the common meaning of the words used (e.g., black holes are not actually coloured black; they are celestial objects that absorb all surrounding matter and energy within a certain proximity, therefore, they emit no light and do not have a colour; and black holes are not actually holes, just extremely dense objects).[6]

If you think about everything you know, it's a lot. Every person you've ever known, every activity, every sight and sound. The fact that all this knowledge is already there in your brain makes acquiring new information, new knowledge, much easier. New knowledge doesn't have to start afresh – rather, it connects up with your existing knowledge. If you already know that planets are spherical, it is easier for you to understand that the Earth is too. If you already know all about Stormzy, you will more readily get Dave. If you have the idea of what 'parts per million' is from reading about carbon dioxide pollution, applying the same to methane is a doddle. The knowledge already in your brain makes it more likely for new information to stick – it makes learning much more efficient. There's a paradox here for teachers: to what extent do you exploit novelty – to make learning interesting, or exploit familiarity – because it's easier to learn when it connects to existing knowledge? As with many aspects of expert teaching, the optimal approach involves finding a balance and tuning it to individual student needs.

6   For astrophysics aficionados: https://www.forbes.com/sites/startswithabang/ 2019/07/10/sorry-black-holes-arent-actually-black/, and https://www. sciencefocus.com/space/is-a-black-hole-a-hole/.

Knowledge is handled in brain systems which are specialists in different domains – the visual system deals with visual information, the auditory system with auditory information. The long-term knowledge of these systems is stored, as with all brain systems, in the strength of their connections. If all these systems were just firing away willy-nilly, with no direction, there would be constant, overwhelming, brain cacophony. To bring some kind of order, coordinating and controlling these systems, there needs to be another system: it's called the modulatory system and we met it back in Chapter 2. Psychologists often refer to this system as the 'executive control' system and that's quite a useful term here; the metaphor of an organisation which has someone (the executive) in charge, who has the power to put plans and action into effect but who has only limited knowledge of the work on the factory floor, conveys the right sense of this system. It has connections to all the other systems, a finger in every pie, and it is very goal-oriented. It activates the parts of the systems that it needs for a particular goal and it inhibits those systems which are not needed or which are superfluous. It prepares the brain to carry out a set of tasks, oriented to the goal; it switches between sub-tasks within that goal when it needs to; and it keeps track of the steps involved, accounting for where it is on the to-do list. It also keeps an eye out for any external influences which might affect the plan so it is ready to change tack if it needs to.

The modulatory or executive system sits at the front of the brain – it's the main reason we humans have bigger foreheads than most of our evolutionary ancestors who are less adept at making dinner plans. And remember the front of the cortex is connected throughout to the limbic system, so our emotions have a direct say in where our attention is pointed, which systems become activated and which are switched to silent. The executive system does not have knowledge as such – it can't actually operate any of the machines on the factory floor. That's why it's called an executive – it doesn't get bogged down in the detail. Its speciality is control, plain and simple.

An everyday example, probably familiar to everyone, illustrates this: have you ever walked upstairs to get something, then got upstairs only to realise you've forgotten what you went up for? (If you haven't had this feeling, you either have a perfect brain or you live in a bungalow.) What's happening is the executive system is keeping the plan – go upstairs to retrieve item – active, but it has lost contact with the specialised system which holds the content of that plan – what the item is and where to find it. The executive can search as hard as it likes for the content but it isn't there – unless it can remake the connection. Sometimes, going back to the place where the plan was made helps restore this connection because it re-engages the sensory system which led to it – you go back downstairs and see that there's no loo roll. Bingo.

THINKING NEEDS MEMORY

We have talked about the substrate for thinking a little and now we'll go in a bit deeper. All the input from our senses offers a lot for the brain to work with – but the brain does not just operate in the here and now. It also draws on all our previous sensory input and our interpretation of it, that is, our memory. Thinking is a cocktail of present and past. In the next sections, we will consider what remembering is for the brain.

A WORD ON TERMINOLOGY

Getting neuroscientists and psychologists and clinicians to agree on a taxonomy of memory has been a failure. Unfortunately, this means there is some pretty ghastly language around memory. Many words used to describe types of memory are really hard to remember. Design flaw! There are also just a lot of terms, used differently by different groups. You might have heard of long-term, short-term, sensory and working memory. Or procedural, declarative, autobiographical, contextual or semantic memory. Explicit and implicit memory. It can be overwhelming. Here we will try to keep the terminology to a minimum. We will instead concentrate on what the needs of different memory systems are and how they work. In the meantime, for those taxonomy fans, here's the main gist (Figure 5.2).

Essentially, there are three types of memory we will be concerned with here: (1) memory for specific things or events (what my Mum was wearing yesterday, how sick I felt when I got my A level results – we have referred to these before as 'instances'); (2) memory for general facts and information, often when we need the gist rather than specifics (countries have borders, what dogs

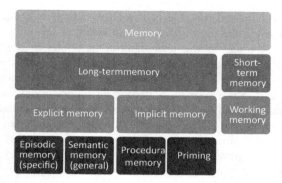

Figure 5.2 The taxonomy of memory and its various components

look like, P is a letter in the alphabet); and (3) memory for how to physically do things (drive a car, tie a tie, write, read). These are all types of long-term memory. In Chapter 6, which is all about learning, we will also talk about a type of short-term memory called working memory – which you can think of as a kind of 'shopping list' memory – you need to keep 'eggs', 'sugar' and 'a lettuce' jiggling away in your mind for long enough to get to the shop, tick off the items as you put them in the basket, then you can throw that mental list away.[7] For now, we are chiefly concerned with memories that stay longer than that.

Generally, when you remember anything, you tie together a lot of connected aspects of that thing. Let's say you saw a bright flash in the sky – you don't just remember 'lightning', you remember how it looked, its shape, whether there were sounds associated with it, maybe where you were when you first saw it, how it made you feel. These links between your different senses and emotions are like the lines in a constellation of stars, ties which together map out 'lightning'. Your lightning constellation is unique, made up of your unique senses and emotions. Someone else's will be different. But tying different people's similar constellations together with the word 'lightning' allows us to communicate about it.

7   One thing all types of memory have in common is that they are not passive. Memory is *active*, rebuilt each time and sensitive to context. We will see some of the implications of this in Chapter 6.

We've mentioned the role of the hippocampus in memory and hopefully got across the slightly abstruse idea that although memory itself doesn't reside in the hippocampus (it resides in the cortex), without the hippocampus you cannot link the different memory ingredients together. To slightly caricature it, think of the memory that Paddington is a bear from Peru. The hippocampus makes the connection between bear and Peru and Paddington – but the individual bits of information – of Paddington and bear and Peru – reside in the cortex. Sometimes when we forget things, we feel that we 'know that we know' something but can't find the memory; usually the reason is that the connection has been lost. The hippocampus serves this binding role in the early days of a memory but does not do it permanently; it typically plays the binding role for about three months. During this time, the job is gradually being handed over (by which we mean played and replayed as described earlier) to the cortex. The cortex is a tortoise – it takes a long time to slowly change its connections and take over the binding that connects memories. One pathological implication of this is that injury to the hippocampus damages knowledge acquired in the last three months but not further back.

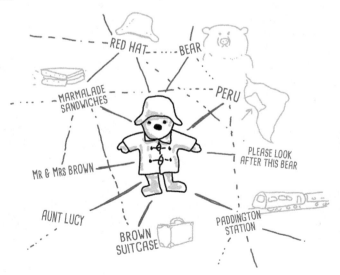

Different types of memory perform different functions so they need different treatment. When it comes to remembering my Gran's 80th birthday party, I want the specifics, the detail, where it was, who was there, what I wore, what my stylish cousin wore, what the funny joke was that Gran told in her speech. But when it comes to remembering the capital of Sierra Leone is Freetown, I don't want to remember the page of the map it was on, or what the weather was like the day I found that out.

Finally, there's the sort of memory I need that allows me to tie my shoelaces in the morning without having to laboriously make a loop and take the dog for a walk around an imaginary pond – the memory of practised, usually physical procedures.

These are very different requirements: the first demands a snapshot of all the sensory and emotional experiences of an event brought together, the second requires the extraction of a single key fact from a sea of irrelevance, and the third needs an automated programme. How does the brain achieve these various memory feats? Answer: With different memory systems. Let's go.

SPECIFIC MEMORIES

Memory of specific episodes melds content with context. Memories here must not be muddled up with other similar memories. We want them to be kept distinct. We don't want to know generally speaking what an 80th birthday party is like; we want to know exactly what Gran's was like. This kind of memory also has to be made quickly. There is no opportunity for a gradual accumulation of experience, this is a one-time thing. But as with all memory formation, that doesn't mean that there is a single place where the whole memory resides as a lump; the memory is made up of a whole array of sensory experiences brought together through specific connections.

This type of memory is typically rich in emotional content, in a way that factual memory generally isn't. Forming these memories is dependent on an additional part of the emotional system which we met in Chapter 3: the amygdala, best known for its role in the 'fight or flight' response. It's clear why our brains should be highly adapted to remember frightening things; matters of survival are top of the priority list for the brain. Remembering everything about a situation when we encountered a frightening event or person is important – where did it happen, what time of day, who else was there – and memories of such events will be laid down strongly and permanently. The idea is simple: recognise the situation where the bad thing happened so that you are better prepared next time.

New research is showing that the amygdala has a much more varied role than just responding to fear, anxiety and threat. It is also important for forming positive memories, such as memories of events that resulted in some kind of reward. The evolving picture of the amygdala is that its business is measuring up the emotional importance of things in the environment – are they good or bad for us? – and generating an emotional response to the important ones. It is also involved in storing memories of them. So the amygdala is crucial for the consolidation of memories with a strong emotional component.

These memories, involving awareness of oneself in a particular time and place, are clearly highly individual as well as highly specific. Two people at the same event at the same time will experience it, and so remember it, very differently. As we understand more about the power of emotions in learning, further investigations of how exactly the amygdala works are potentially of great interest to educators. What are the conditions that will trigger a positive response from the amygdala to enhance learning?

GENERAL MEMORIES

The other main type of long-term memory involves memories of facts and information. The way this kind of memory works is quite different. We want to throw out a lot of the extraneous information, lay a lot of different specific experiences down on top of each other and look for common patterns in all of them. We want to remember what, in general, a park is, rather than the specific details of this particular park on this particular day.[8] This more

8   For a fascinating first-hand description of what it is like *not* to pull out the 'gist' in this way, see this wonderful TED talk by Temple Grandin, who was diagnosed with autism as a child and vividly describes how her own memory works: https://www.ted.com/talks/temple_grandin_the_world_needs_all_kinds_of_minds?language=en.

general type of knowledge allows us to deploy our previous experience when we encounter new situations – it is knowledge that is characterised by the fact it can generalise. A piece of this general knowledge – of the number six, of alliteration, of revenge as a motivating force – can be drawn on and deployed in a totally different, new context, as a shortcut. Key to this kind of memory formation is getting to grips with *concepts*.

CONCEPTS AND REPRESENTATIONS

Our brain has a great capacity to form concepts. You see a type of dog you've never seen before but your concept of dog is strong enough that you know this funny-looking one with a missing leg and a squashed face is still a dog. Or you come across an unknown word in a sentence: your concepts of how the letters in a word combine to produce sounds means you can pronounce it, and the context (the rest of the words in the sentence) allows you to have a good stab at this unknown word's meaning. You use your existing concepts to embrace new ones.

Our concepts are not fixed things. Concepts are a shifting set of connected neural activations, recreated each time that concept is evoked. And each time you conjure a concept, those activations will be slightly different. If I ask you to think of a shark, a certain set of connections will be activated. If I say the word *lawyer*, then the word *shark*, a different set will be activated. If I say the word *endangered* and then the word *shark*, a different set again will be activated. The set activated if you think of *shark* at home on your sofa is different from those evoked if you are swimming out of your depth in the sea off Bondi Beach.

When we are learning new concepts, new relevant experiences will be woven into the existing concept memory, subtly changing its shape. Let's say our concept of 'dog' generally involves the idea of benign, tail-wagging four-legged creatures of various shapes and sizes who go for walks attached to people via long pieces of string. Then one day a dog snarls at us and bares its teeth and we are frightened. Not only is the memory of that event stored as a specific snapshot memory with strong emotional content, but the new information about dogs will also be wired into our existing concept, which might shift, so that a 'dog' is now a '*generally* benign' or '*sometimes* benign' or, if we were really affected by the experience, '*invariably malign*' four-legged creature. To move the new knowledge from specific memory into conceptual memory needs sleep: it is during sleep that the brain replays activity in the hippocampus to the cortex which gradually changes its connections in response and integrates it with previous knowledge.[9]

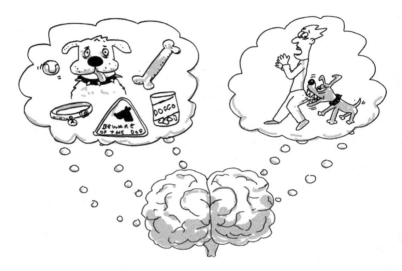

Concepts are an important component of this type of general memory. The home of concepts is the outer layer of the brain: the cortex. As we have seen, this is the place where long-term memories, with help from the hippocampus, are stored. Concepts are an efficient way of bringing together diverse experiences. If we give them a label, usually a word, then that's even more helpful. The word is a shorthand for the concept which allows us to communicate about it. If we think of the word 'jungle', just hearing the word conjures sights and sounds and smells based on every encounter, real or virtual, that we have ever

9   There's a potential danger that replaying a memory to move it might lead to that memory being recorded again – and again, and again! To avoid making multiple memories, we usually don't remember our dreams as new memories, unless we carry on thinking about them after we wake up (so storing them as new awake memories).

had with jungles. Jungles are damp, colourful, exist in certain climates, contain a multitude of flora and fauna, they are noisy with the sounds of animals and potentially contain dangers, such as venomous snakes. They are threatened by human activity and climate change. The word and its concept are a portal to the whole world of knowledge and experience. Even though someone else's concept of 'jungle' will be different, being grounded in their unique set of experiences – there is enough of an overlap to make communication possible.

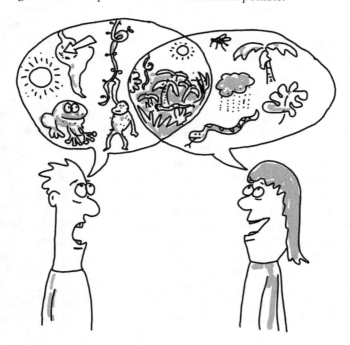

MEMORIES OF HOW TO DO THINGS

The third main type of long-term memory is memory of how to do things. It usually involves our motor systems. Back in Chapter 2 we saw how, with hours of repeated practice, certain actions can become automatic. A toddler starting to use a knife and fork instead of her fingers, a child in reception learning to match shapes and sounds of letters in order to read, a teenager learning to drive a car. These are activities that most of us learned and which are now so automatic that we cannot imagine not doing them – in fact, it is almost impossible to look at letters and *not* read them. The amount of practice required to make these sorts of skills automatic can be huge: tens or hundreds of hours, repeating again and again until all the neural activity is streamlined and fluent. For reading, it is estimated that it takes about 2000 hours of practice for children to become fluent.[10] The cerebellum – remember that little lump at the back of the brain which holds 80 per cent of our neurons? – is an important new addition to memory systems for this kind of motor procedure memory, as are circuits that loop between the cortex and lower levels of the brain, such as the thalamus.

A SHOUT-OUT TO FORGETTING

In the next chapters, we will be dealing with learning, that is, both how we acquire new knowledge and skills and how we remember them well enough to draw on them when we need to. Retention, i.e., maintaining knowledge, retrieval, i.e., finding it, and forgetting, i.e., losing it, will all be crucial to understanding that. For now, we want to acknowledge the important point that even though we often curse ourselves for forgetting things and wish our memories were better, for our memories to work well, they really *need* to forget. Knowing what to forget is almost as important a job for the brain as knowing what to keep.[11] Just imagine if you tried to keep every smell, every sight, every sound, every thought that you have had for your whole life. Overwhelming.

There are two main types of forgetting – the process of instantly throwing away newly acquired information (the colour of the car which passed before you crossed the road, the results from the rugby match in this morning's sports report – assuming you're not into rugby) and the slower decay of memories that have made it to

10 See Thomas, Knowland and Rogers (2020).
11 How the brain goes about this seems to be via the reward system. Experiences which are associated with rewards produce more dopamine. Dopamine seems to 'tag' such memories for intensified reprocessing during sleep, so that the rewarding experiences of the previous day are better remembered, while those without reward are more likely to be forgotten (Asfestani et al., 2020).

long-term memory storage but are not being used. Both of these types of forgetting can be affected by many things – how the knowledge is acquired (e.g., things which are heard are more easily forgotten than things which are read), things going on around that knowledge which change its importance (I'm playing car bingo with my friend so I remember that the car that passed was yellow), how well integrated the knowledge was with existing knowledge, and by time itself. Some knowledge naturally decays quickly, other knowledge decays depending on how much it is used. We'll find out how to minimise forgetting in Chapter 6.

Another type of forgetting is known as confabulation – or what some have called 'telling it like it isn't' (Gilboa & Verfaellie, 2010). As we have seen, long-term memory involves a whole set of connections between different pieces of information distributed widely in the brain – a whole array of facts, emotions, sensory traces. When we think of simple things – Paddington is a bear from Peru – the pathways are clearly defined and we can be 100 per cent accurate in reporting on the result of the memory search. When we deal with more complex and less-used concepts or memories, there are likely to be many pathways involved, some more overgrown than others, and possible alternative routes. In such cases, accuracy is not perfect. We do not keep every element of a particular event (Gran's 80th birthday party) and the parts we do keep are stored in many different areas.

What this means is that when we are retrieving that memory, we might not find everything. If that happens, our brain, rather than leave a gap, takes whatever is closest to the missing part and fabricates the missing detail based on what is most likely. This is called confabulation and it is a completely unconscious process. It is not the same as lying because it is not something we do deliberately. It is more akin to how the brain fills in the blanks in a visual illusion, like 'creating' a white square in Figure 5.3. Given the coordinated chunks missing from each circle, to the brain, it's most likely there's a white square sitting in front of four whole circles, so why not add in the edges?. But with time, the fabricated part can become woven into the memory itself. As the memory is recalled, it includes the altered parts, further strengthening their links. This habit of the brain is

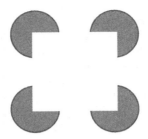

Figure 5.3 There is no white square (discuss)

important for understanding how things can sometimes be *mis-remembered* with great certainty.[12]

DIFFERENCES AND SIMILARITIES

Although we have dwelt on the main differences of different memory systems, there is also much they have in common. They all involve the following set of processes, which we will be using as our framework in Chapter 6 (Figure 5.4).

No matter the system we are talking about, memory is not all neatly in one place, like a folder in a filing cabinet. Rather, all memories involve information that is widely distributed throughout the brain and when memories are recalled, they are reconstructed. It is the links between pieces of information that are key.

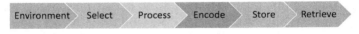

Figure 5.4 From the world to our brain: the stages of memory formation

---

12 If you think you're immune, you should know that no character ever says, 'Play it again, Sam' in *Casablanca*, Darth Vader never says, 'Luke, I am your father' in *Return of the Jedi*, no one says, 'We're going to need a bigger boat' in *Jaws*, Dorothy never says, 'I don't think we're in Kansas any more' in *The Wizard of Oz*. Still confident in your 100 per cent accurate memory? For more, see the masterful film-and-gaming fan site Looper, available at: https://www.looper.com/725660/huge-movie-mandela-effects-thatll-have-you-questioning-everything/.

Memories change with time but different types of memories change differently. While you might well forget the dates of the Impressionist painters, you are very unlikely to forget that you are scared of snakes.[13] A great deal of everyday information is never even encoded so never makes it far along the memory chain.

A completely unfamiliar *experience* is especially easy to remember but a completely unfamiliar *piece of information* is especially hard. If I ask you to remember that 'the pisiform, the lunate and the triquetrum are all on the side of the ulna' or the sentence 'She so extra, tryna flex all over finsta today', you might struggle – these words might have little to hook onto.[14] The hardest thing about forming this kind of memory is embedding new knowledge into the surer systems of existing knowledge – so a completely unfamiliar piece of information presents the greatest challenge. By contrast, for personal memories of events, the hardest thing is keeping each memory clearly defined and distinct from other similar ones – so a completely unfamiliar experience is helpful in offering clearer boundaries.

THINKING ABOUT THINKING

We've seen that, given a choice, the brain would rather stick to the concrete world than operate in the abstract one. To do abstraction, it needs training, it needs executive control, and it needs a lot of practice. Even then, abstract thinking remains founded on sensorimotor experience and emotions. The brain's normal mode of operation is not logical. In fact, humans did OK for hundreds of thousands of years before logic was even invented![15] The brain is not naturally neat

13 It takes many hours with a therapist to overwrite a phobia; desensitisation therapy involves exposure to sufficient instances of <snake + not scary>, for this association to overwrite the amygdala memory of <snake = scary>. The aim is to overwrite the phobic memory with another non-phobic one within the amygdala. Amygdala doesn't forget. Bad memories have to be deliberately overwritten to convince you that you need not fear snakes.

14 We kid you not: The pisiform, lunate and triquetrum are all bones in the wrist. The second sentence might roughly translate as 'She's going crazy showing off all over her fake Instagram account today.'

15 Logical reasoning is a special taught skill that seems to involve inhibitory control to focus on the structures and operations of an argument, usually indicated by its linguistic structure, rather than content and meaning: what

and rule-abiding. It is heavily influenced by what is familiar or probable, it's likely to succumb to peer pressure and it's very affected by potential rewards or losses. It gets tired. It wants soothing repetition like a baby does. It wants a pat on the head.

Nonetheless, we have seen how the brain can do thinking – with the right training and practice, it can reason, understand concepts, solve problems, create. Our thinking can vary in response to encountering different challenges – the sort of thinking we need to do to break up a playground brawl is different from the thinking to plan an event or learn a language or address a philosophical question.

And there is a final piece of the puzzle, which is *thinking about our thinking*, sometimes called *metacognition*. It's one thing to do all our different kinds of thinking but quite another to know we are doing them – and maybe even think about doing them differently. Metacognition describes monitoring our thought processes as they are happening, in real time. Once we have become accustomed to doing this, we might be able to use particular metacognitive strategies to optimise our thought processes for particular types of challenge. These sorts of strategies can entail very simple actions. For example, asking ourselves the simple question, 'Is this thought process working for this particular challenge?' might be enough to prompt a change of thinking approach.

Just as our brains have to be taught and coaxed into engaging in abstract thought, they have to be coaxed and instructed into metacognition. This sort of thinking about thinking is not what we tend naturally to do. But this 'bird's-eye view' of our brain and what it is up to is a potentially fruitful target for successful transfer of learning, that is, to apply what we have learned in one situation to another. It is one of many approaches we will discuss in Chapter 6 as we come to the crux of the educational question: how does the brain learn?

logically follows from the propositions rather than what is probably true. Which is maybe why winning a logical argument can sometimes feel a bit of a Pyrrhic victory (Houdé & Borst, 2015).

LEARNING IS EVEN HARDER

INTRODUCTION

Using our understanding of the brain to improve learning is what educational neuroscience is all about. Sometimes this new perspective
confirms what teachers already know from experience. Sometimes it
shows how current practice might be adjusted to better suit the brain.
Sometimes it highlights areas where we don't yet fully understand the
underlying mechanisms. It's early days for the field of educational
neuroscience.

Learning presents a bit of a contradiction. On the one hand,
the brain *can't help but* learn – it's what it does. On any given day,
whether inside or outside the context of education, the brain is
constantly learning, interpreting sensory input against existing
knowledge, and recording experiences. On the other hand,
deliberate focused learning is hard. No fewer than eight different
brain systems are involved and need to work together. These
include different memory systems – a speedy one for short-term
'snapshots', a slower one for concepts, an emotional system
which maintains associations and helps spur or deter, a control
system to activate appropriate specific content, a dopamine-based
system which responds to the presence or absence of rewards, a
slow-to-perfect system for learning motor procedures such as
doing joined-up writing, a social system that learns through
watching other people, and a language system which allows
learning to happen through verbal instruction. Each has a preferred diet of experience that will optimise its learning. All of this
must be seen in the context of what we now know about the

DOI: 10.4324/9781003185642-6

brain's priorities – senses and movement, emotions (especially motivation) and other people.

Learning involves acquiring and retaining information and being able to retrieve it for future use. There is (sadly!) no 'plug-in' programme for learning a given skill – the brain needs to work out the programme for itself, on the basis of the situations it encounters. Mostly, learning is not a matter of just remembering specific moments. Rather, each situation gives only a partial version of the whole, and the brain will need many exposures that it can overlay to pull out the common themes. The brain also needs to be flexible, so that skills or concepts can be applied in different contexts – again, this takes time, repetition and exposure to varieties of information – as well as usually needing external help to point out how to apply what it has learned to a novel situation.

How well we retain information varies depending on the environment, the timeframe of taking information in, our mood and the method by which the information is taught. How well we retrieve it is similarly affected by the retrieval cues we are given, by our mood, by the context of retrieval and by how the memories themselves have been stored – people vary greatly in how quickly and how well they can form and retrieve memories.

The good news is that we know more and more about how to exploit the systems involved to optimise learning. In Chapter 7, we will be outlining the theory and practice of some of those methods.

FROM ACCESSIBLE IN THE ENVIRONMENT TO ACCESSIBLE IN LONG-TERM MEMORY

When we learn, how do we select what, from all the possible information out there, we want to process? And once we have decided, how do we keep the information active long enough for it to be encoded? What are the requirements of the different memory systems? Once stored, how do we recognise the need to deploy our memories and retrieve them on demand? Let's look once more at the sequence of stages of memory formation (Figure 6.1).

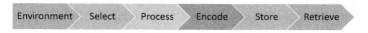

Figure 6.1 From the world to our brain: the stages of memory formation revisited

If we take an example from a classroom setting, imagine a child listening to the teacher explaining how to subtract numbers. The environment is filled with stimuli – the sound of the words, peripheral noises, visual stimuli – other people, the classroom walls, the teacher's red dress, maybe the smell of lunch being cooked or the feel of a new itchy jumper on the skin. From all these stimuli, the first task, which requires attention processes, is to identify and home in on the salient stimulus in order to process and remember it. The second is to discard the rest and forget them. Some of the attended part will engage the modulatory system in keeping this information active in the relevant content systems, such as phonological circuits or visuo-spatial circuits – what is sometimes called working memory. With a bit of luck, it is one of the relevant bits – the words of the teacher saying that 'sub-traction means the same as taking away' or visualising the example of '6 - 4' or processing the meaning of the principle that 'subtraction is like addition in reverse'. With rehearsal, the information can start to be consolidated in the connections of the content systems, and path-ways established to retrieve and reactivate it on cue, that is, from long-term memory. Over time and with practice and repetition, it will become more firmly established in long-term memory so that it can be retrieved, for example, in a maths lesson later on in the week.

We'll take each of these stages in turn.

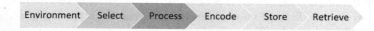

SELECTION AND PROCESSING

ATTENTION

We know from earlier chapters that the brain is a very active organ, constantly making predictions about what is going to happen. It is *always* paying attention. It just might not be paying attention to the thing that it is 'meant' to be attending to.

From an evolutionary perspective, attention is a tool to direct our sensory systems to the information our motor system needs to pro-duce a response – visually orienting to a fly in order to lash out our tongue or turning our head in response to a yelp from a parent. In that context, the goal is very clear and drives the attention in a way that is highly directed to that goal. Attention is a filter to select information from the environment – the all-important first step in the learning cascade (Posner & Rothbart, 2014). If the information does not make it past the front door, it can't get processed. Many educational goals, such as problem-solving, reasoning, analysing, critical thinking, creativity, involve higher-level processes. But to improve them, we first need to be sure that attention is working well (Amso & Scerif, 2015).

Attention is sometimes described in terms of levels: at the bottom is the 'alerting' system which is a state of awakened readiness brought about by something unexpected in the environment. Next up is the 'orienting' system, particularly important in infants and very young children, which points our attention to the right stimulus; it might operate automatically – for example, when we hear a loud bang or see a flashing light – or voluntarily – for example, when we look away from something which we find disturbing. By the time we reach mid-childhood, control of attention is mainly the job of the executive, modulatory network, which, as we saw in earlier chapters, works in cahoots with emotion systems to set priorities and goals for the sensorimotor systems.

Whichever level we consider, attention can be thought of as a computation which is applied to competing information from the environment (listen to the teacher or my whispering neighbour) or from abstract, internal information sources (such as competing goals: should I stay or should I go?). The result of the competition is that certain information 'wins' and is selected, while the alternatives lose and are filtered out. This filtering can operate in a specific sensory domain (I notice the sound of someone's voice; you notice the colour of their eyes) or more abstractly (from my mental list of chores, I focus on clearing out the kitchen cupboards).

When the brain attends to something, connections between the executive control system and the hippocampus are activated. In laboratory tests where participants are asked to 'think about' one set of stimuli and 'not think about' another set, clear differences can be seen in the activation of the hippocampus – that is, when the brain is 'not thinking', the normally active hippocampus becomes less active. It's the executive network's way of signalling to the brain's storage system that something important is coming down the track (Posner & Rothbart, 2014).

Many things can get in the way of attention in the classroom. There are external sources of distraction – noise, eye-catching visual displays, technology, as well as internal ones such as mind wandering. We'll talk later about how to help minimise those.

WORKING MEMORY

Sensory memory is very short-lived – neurons will typically continue to fire for about a quarter of a second after experiencing a sensory stimulus. To do anything useful with the contents, there needs to be some way of keeping the content activated for longer. If a particular sensory stimulus has 'won' the attention computation, that information will now be handled by what is commonly referred to as 'working memory'. The term 'working memory' has been used by cognitive psychologists for many years and some unhelpful concepts and language have accumulated around it – all connected to the idea of working memory being a sort of transient 'memory box'. The idea of such a memory box pretty clearly contravenes everything we have said so far about how the brain works! Working memory should rather be thought of as the establishment of temporary links from the executive system at the front of the brain to the sensory circuits, which then keep the sensory circuits active *even in the absence of the sensory input*. A classic working memory-involving scenario could be repeating a phone number again and again in your head once the numbers on a screen are no longer available to your eyes. Working memory is the active maintenance of a set of neuronal connections which are vulnerable (if someone shouts your name as you are mentally rehearsing that phone number, it's gone), of limited duration (imagine 10 minutes of repeating the phone number – too exhausting to manage unless there's something huge at stake) and with limited capacity (if it's a 20-digit phone number, you're probably not even going to attempt it).[1]

1   This capacity issue is something of a mystery to neuroscientists (Gabi et al., 2016). The prefrontal cortex has over a billion neurons, which seems enough to handle even a really long phone number.

The concept of a 'task set' which we introduced in Chapter 2 is relevant here. A task set, you'll remember, is a formula involving all the sensory and motor components needed for a specific task. Think of whack-a-mole. A task set is, 'See a mole pop out of a hole: hit it with a mallet.' An alternative task set might be, 'See a bunny pop out of a hole: do not hit it.' The basic neuroscience (worked out with cooperative monkeys and not involving moles or mallets) required monkeys to perform something known as a 'match to sample' task: keep stimulus A in mind when it disappears from view, then respond to say whether stimulus B, which appears in view, is the same or different from A. To complete this task, what is required is not the 'storage' of information about task A but rather the real-time activation of the links from sensory circuits to the frontal cortex to keep the sensory information alive even once it has disappeared from the environment. It is a crucial difference between passive storage and active maintenance of neuronal connections. Seen like this, it is hopefully clear that it will be highly influenced by the mode (is it words, a visual stimulus, a mental map), by the current environment (how clearly defined it is from competing sensory input), as well as by the in-the-moment contribution of motivation and reward.

Working memory can be thought of as a sort of wipe-clean whiteboard − information can be maintained there for a limited period of time before it is wiped off, usually to be replaced by something else. There are limits to capacity, but what defines capacity is variable − to extend the whiteboard metaphor: How big is the writing? Are there different coloured pens used? Are the words interesting or banal? Are there pictures as well as words? And even more broadly, Am I tired or cross or just can't be bothered to look at it? Do my friends seem interested? The metaphor is imperfect in that, as we have seen, the whiteboard of working memory is distributed throughout other systems (the content) while the 'keep it active' element is a common mechanism with no writing on. In terms of what is happening in the brain, working memory means keeping a pattern of neurons firing for long enough that their output can be used. When I am working out what 6^3 is in my head, I am using working memory to keep the stages of my calculation on my mental whiteboard. Six sixes are thirty six ... now, times *that* by six... It is a place for the *conscious, active* processing of information. Information cannot secretly be in working memory.

A common psychological model of working memory is made up of three components: (1) a central executive (the overall manager, with links to long-term memory); (2) a visual storage system (the 'visuospatial sketchpad' – a mental picture of the contents); and (3) a verbal storage system: the 'phonological loop' – the voice in our head (Baddeley, 2003). If the contents of working memory are rehearsed through the visual or auditory system (think of repeating the shopping list to yourself as you walk to the shop), they are more likely to be stored in long-term memory.

Let's take a simple example to illustrate what we mean by the rather convoluted idea that working memory capacity is limited and yet variable. It seems that working memory can handle about seven gobbets of information. We use the word 'gobbet' deliberately to draw attention to the messy answer to the question of what the contents of that information might be. Look at these numbers:

100365246060

Now cover them up and see if you can remember them. How did you do? Most people won't be able to manage them all.

How about if we write them like this?

100 365 24 60 60

Does that help?

How about if I tell you that these are the numbers of years in a century, the number of days in a year, the number of hours in a day, the number of minutes in an hour and the number of seconds in a minute?

Generally, this extra information will make the process of remembering much much easier. This process is called 'chunking' and refers to the fact that although the gobbets of information that can be held in working memory seems to be limited to about seven (about the same as parrots are capable of), the overall amount of information is much greater than that suggests. It depends on how it is presented, prior knowledge, be botheredness and more.

So working memory is the temporary maintenance of a dynamic pattern of neural firing. How does that help us? Well, the simplest implication is that, notwithstanding the variability, there are some limits to what we can take on board in any one go; we can't keep up the firing of an indeterminate number of neurons indefinitely. If I expect my class to learn at a stroke the ten wonders of the world, I might have trouble. Particularly early on in a learning journey, less is usually more.

Now the next important question is whether items have sufficiently aroused the interest of the frontal cortex so that, given the goal, their activity should be maintained back in the relevant content systems. The longer the activations are sustained, the more likely that those sensory systems will alter in response, that hippocampus will record the event and that PFC-sensory cortex connections will strengthen – and the memory cascade is under way. Our pyramid of priorities is useful here because the likelihood of items being stored is in relation to where they are on that pyramid. Things which affect our survival will almost certainly be quickly stored, since evolution – specifically, natural selection – had a lot to work on there. Strongly emotional experiences, whether good or bad, are also likely to be stored permanently, because they are the brain's way of maximising the chances it will get what it wants next time. Beyond that, what is stored is dependent on what makes sense and has meaning for the individual (Sousa, 2011). Let's look once more at the brain's priorities (Figure 6.2).

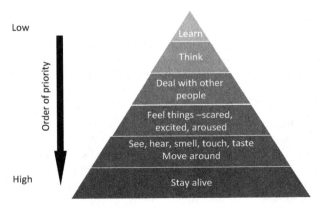

Figure 6.2 The brain's priorities also influence which memories are stored

Whether information makes sense and has meaning has to do with past experience – since both understanding (making sense of something) and finding meaning (seeing the relevance of it) are concerned with how this new knowledge connects to previous knowledge and experience. Knowledge that is both understandable and relevant has the best chance of being stored.[2] Of the two criteria, meaning seems to have the greater impact on what is stored. This is illustrated daily in classrooms, where children are able to apply a new piece of learning – a new maths technique, a device for beginning a story – in the moment but the next day they cannot remember what to do. Usually this is because the new content made sense but lacked meaning. For teachers, it is as important to think 'how can I help make this meaningful for students, given their past experience?' as it is to think 'how can I help them understand it?' (Sousa, 2011). As we will see, one way that knowledge can be given more meaning is by connecting it to other, seemingly unrelated knowledge. Emotional connections are also likely to make for stronger tethers to storage systems.

A FEW WORDS ON COGNITIVE LOAD THEORY

There has been much discussion in recent years about 'cognitive load theory', with some big claims[3] about its importance to educators. The idea is that the 'cognitive load' involved in a task is the amount of information processing required to perform it. The load is made up of different types of loads: (1) *intrinsic load* – how hard something is, which will depend on previous knowledge; (2) *extraneous load* – other information processing connected with how information is delivered; and (3) *germane load* – elements that aid processing. The theory, in a nutshell, is that if the cognitive load exceeds the processing capacity of the learner, they won't learn it.

The theory undoubtedly has positive aspects – the key one being to promote the idea that to be successful, teaching must be at an appropriate level of challenge. Too much means it is hard to

---

2   There are subtleties to what is going on; events that conform to our expectations are better remembered than unrelated events but events that *conflict* can also be remembered better depending on what information is being sought at recall (Greve et al., 2019).

3   See https://twitter.com/dylanwiliam/status/824682504602943489?lang=en

process, since there are insufficient hooks to previous knowledge; too little means boredom. There is also the idea that intrinsic load can be high, if there are no links to long-term memory, for example, if a completely new subject area is presented without context or analogies and that extrinsic load can be high, if the information is presented badly, with key information and extraneous irrelevant or non-crucial information combined, or distracting features which deflect from the key information. All these elements are reasonable.

Based on what we have learned about the brain, the problem with how the theory is sometimes presented is that it positions the brain as an inert device into which external input is poured, filling it up like water in a bucket. If the bucket is full, no more water can get in. In fact, a better analogy for the brain is more a whole water supply chain, devices filling and emptying at varying speeds and rates of spillage depending on whether there's an imminent flood, whether it's just a game, or a high-stakes competition, whether the task is enjoyable, whether our friends are also part of the chain – and sometimes the system demands more water because it's thirsty.

The issue then is one of emphasis: cognitive load theory puts all the emphasis on thinking as if it is a separable element of what the brain does; it puts the emphasis on teacher-led rather than student-led learning and downplays social and subjective elements of learning. The key point is that there is a lot more to processing than 'space in working memory'. There are all sorts of reasons why students might not take in information – they are not interested, they have low self-esteem, they don't get on with the teacher, they are hungry – which are highly individual and highly variable. The idea of 'cognitive load' is appealing because it suggests something eminently measurable – weighable even! – but there are no established measures for it. It also does not address how children's thinking skills change with age, particularly with respect to executive function skills. It instead focuses on changes in prior knowledge as the key age-related change. In fact, we know that

Environment   Select   Process   Encode   Store   Retrieve

encoding and retrieval are performed better by a more mature executive function system.[4]

ENCODING AND STORAGE

The basic process of storing memories was described in Chapter 5. It involves the interplay between the hippocampus (which encodes the information) and the cortex (where it is stored), it takes time and it requires sleep. The first 24 hours are quite a useful guide to retention, since the majority of loss of newly acquired knowledge happens in the first 18–24 hours after acquisition. If it's not there after 24 hours, it's unlikely that it has been stored (Sousa, 2011). Long-term memory, we cannot emphasise enough, is not a filing cabinet with a neat label; it is a constantly shifting, interactive system which activates areas all over the brain to retrieve and rebuild what we call memories. Memories are not bricks; they are jelly.

Although we have talked about memory systems already, we want to take a moment to go into a bit more detail about what a memory is at the brain cell level. Picturing this will help understand the strengths and weaknesses of the system – and potentially offer up fruitful ways to intervene in it. It all starts when nerve impulses from sensory neurons, in response to a stimulus (the smell of a rose, the colour of a felt tip, the letter Q) cause a neuron to fire – to send out an electrical signal. If the signal is strong enough, it will cause an adjacent neuron, connected to it, to fire as well, and in turn stimulate other neurons to fire. The group of neurons that fire in response to that signal comprise the memory-set for that particular thing. Sometimes the firing does not last for long and the memory (that is, the firing of that group of neurons) is lost. Though even without the initial firing, neurons will stay in a ready state – where they need a lower level of stimulation to fire – for several hours. Psychologists call this effect 'priming'. Such an event results in what we might call a fleeting perception, the sense of a thing, a temporary neural trace.

At other times, the firing continues for longer, and a pattern of repeated firing is set up. The faster a neuron fires, the bigger its

---

4   For more on this, as well as other great resources from the Research Schools Network, see https://researchschool.org.uk/huntington/news and https://researchschool.org.uk/

electrical signal and the more likely it is to set off its neighbours. As this happens repeatedly, parts of the surface of the neurons change so that they are sensitised, that is, they become more likely to fire again in response to the signal from the connecting neuron. Eventually, the activity of this repeating firing patterns binds the neurons more and more closely to each other, until they work as a firing team. When one fires, they all fire – 'Neurons that fire together wire together'[5] – and a new memory is made. Clusters of these sort of memory traces form networks, so that when one is activated, the whole network gets strengthened. When we are prompted by something that touches on one part of the network, the whole network will become activated – as when a single smell can bring a cascade of memories flooding back. The parts of these memories are spread out all over the brain. Even the simplest memory is distributed widely; an orange in memory means the colour of it in one place, the feel of it in another, the smell somewhere else. These are physically far apart: as we have seen, the different sensory systems lie in different lobes in the back of the brain. All these networks are brought together by the simple thought of an orange.

This should help us visualise why new knowledge is easier to acquire when it is founded on existing knowledge. Rather than having to build a whole new network from scratch, the new knowledge simply piggybacks on existing knowledge, using its more firmly established set-up. When we use memory tricks like remembering someone's name by associating it with something else that is familiar – Rose rhymes with nose or picturing a rose when we picture the person Rose – that is what we are doing: strapping new knowledge onto the firm trunk of existing knowledge. The more connections we can make, the more meaning can be attached to new knowledge. And also the more likely the memory is to be stored in many different areas – which is very useful for retrieving the information, as there are many different routes to accessing it. We will see later how this has practical applications for the classroom.

We have talked about encoding and storage in general terms but, as we saw in Chapter 5, there are several different memory systems, each with unique requirements. *Specific* memories of

5   This phrase was coined by Donald Hebb in 1949, to describe how brain pathways are formed and strengthened by repetition.

episodes in my life – what I wore yesterday, who came to my birthday party – need to store different things from *general* memories concerning facts and less personalised knowledge – the longest river in the world, the titles of Amanda Gorman poems, the number 3. And both of those have different requirements from memory of how to do things – read a book, tie a tie.

Specific memories rely on the hippocampus and amygdala and this system changes its connections very quickly. It needs to, in order to record snapshots in the moment, to capture the here and now. For the general system, associations between knowledge, perceptual information and motor responses must be learnt. This involves, as we have seen in earlier chapters, spotting complex patterns within the knowledge – complex patterns we call concepts – a job for the cortex. This process is very slow; changing connections in the cortex takes many hours, it requires repetition of experiences and may need variable instances of the concepts to understand their scope and the contexts in which they are found, very different from 'one-shot' learning.

The system for procedures works through sheer slog – of repeating the activity (whether it is reading or tying ties) for many many hours – hundreds of hours – until it becomes automatic and we can 'do it without thinking about it'. This mostly means not having to bother the frontal cortex, the modulatory (executive) system, which has notoriously limited capacity, so better to leave it be when you can to get on with something else. These procedural activities also depend on the cortex but here cortical connections are to brain regions distinct from other memory systems – the basal ganglia, the thalamus, and the cerebellum.

There's another type of memory system that we don't even think of as a memory system because it is implicit. We know that when the bell goes, it's time for break. We avoid Brussel sprouts because we hate the taste. We have learned these associations through conditioning. This is the classic 'Pavlovian' response where something (the stimulus) comes to be associated with a particular response – those dogs salivating when the bell rings is the brain in full autopilot mode.

Finally we should mention a type of memory that we think about even less. Have you ever wondered why you don't spend the whole day processing the feeling of your socks on your feet (unless there's a hole in the toe)? This is a different kind of learning called habituation – it is learning to ignore. It is the brain adjusting to the

environment and screening out unimportant information – the feel of
our socks, the sound of our breathing – to focus on what is important.

REHEARSAL

Making sense of new learning takes time – to process and reprocess
the information, often several times. For learning that involves
motor skills (tying that tie) we call this *practice*, and for information
processing, we call it *rehearsal*. If you've repeated a phone number
to yourself several times to help remember it, that's rehearsal. It
typically first happens when the information engages working
memory and involves the frontal cortex – the executive system.
The speed of processing varies a great deal from person to person.
Similarly, the next stages of processing happen at different rates for
different people and for different content and contexts.

There are various types of rehearsal. The simplest is the sort of rote
rehearsal we associate with learning times tables, or a poem we are to
recite, or the steps of a recipe. Elaborative rehearsal is more complex and
involves the fleshing out of knowledge. While rote rehearsal is something many people do without being taught (repeating the list of who is
coming to your party as you write the invites), elaborative rehearsal
usually has to be taught. It is less the brute force hammering of rote
rehearsal and more the fine needlepoint of making connections
between new knowledge and existing knowledge. Rather than being
the rehearsal of the lyrics of a song, it is the rehearsal of the lyrics' tex-
tures, meanings, and interpretations. It is not 6 x 5 = 30, it is understanding why 6 x 5 is the same as 5 x 6. The more someone finds
meaning in the new information, a process which might take time, the
more likely they are to retain it. Elaboration is a deliberate, and often
difficult, activity.

Later in the chapter we will talk about other factors which affect
how well information is retained, including when it is taught (e.g., in a
sequence, the first and the last parts are likely to be best retained), how
long the teaching block is (e.g., retention will be better in 2 x 20-
minute blocks than the same information in a single 40-minute one),

Environment   Select   Process   Encode   Store   Retrieve

how long there is between blocks of learning and how the information is taught (lectures don't do well here!).

RETRIEVAL

The final step in effective learning is being able to retrieve a stored memory when we need to. We can do this by recognition – matching up an external stimulus with information we have stored: the correct spelling of a word from a list of choices, the actor who was in a film we saw last year – or we can do it by recall. Recall involves sending out a search cue to long-term memory – something that can reawaken the memory item and enable working memory to reactivate the relevant content in conceptual and sensory systems. The act of retrieving, enabling working memory to reactivate information within long-term memory systems, means relearning it, which is why retrieval practice is such an important and useful classroom practice (we'll talk about ways to make it most effective later in Chapter 7).

There are several things which affect the rate and effectiveness of memory retrieval. Context is a very important one: recall is much more likely to be accurate if the context in which a memory is being retrieved closely resembles the context of information storage. If we can't recall something, but then return to the place we originally thought about it – bingo! – in that memory pops: that's context at work (Cottingham, n.d.). How good the search cue is also affects retrieval. The act of remembering is very active – it is not about 'finding a thing' so much as 'rebuilding a thing', since memories must be reconstructed each time within the content systems that originally processed the information. This process is made easier if the cue is a strong trigger for the reconstruction. Also, as we mentioned in the last section, elaborative rehearsal provides more entry points for memory access. If these strong links have been built between the executive system and the memory storage systems, which enables working memory to reactivate the information, this too facilitates retrieval.

A final important point about retrieval is that it varies a great deal from person to person – not just because of differences in processing speed, but because of the fundamental structure of memories. Memory formation involves linking new knowledge to our existing knowledge based on previous experience: clearly that is highly individual. This means that for each of us, our memories are distributed across different networks, and retrieval rates vary depending on the networks they are stored in. Conceptual knowledge, as we've mentioned, needs to be encountered in many contexts, to help spot the overlaps that together represent that concept. The fewer the contexts, the more likely the knowledge is to be subject to the idiosyncrasies of an individual's experience – and the more variable the ease of access.

All this makes the process of retrieval faster for some than others – an important consideration in the classroom, where speed is sometimes king. It is also important (and perhaps surprising) that the rate of retrieval (getting items out or reactivating items within long-term memory) is quite distinct from the rate of learning (putting them in or encoding them within its structure). Some people who learn quickly take a long time to retrieve the knowledge and vice versa. This is important in the context of education since timed tests are so prevalent and these take the speed of retrieving answers to be a key metric by which to judge learning. The good news is that there are many techniques that can be taught to better gear long-term memory storage to fast and effective retrieval; we'll be coming to them in Chapter 7.

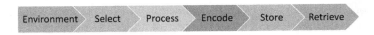

Environment   Select   Process   Encode   Store   Retrieve

We have made it to the end of the memory cycle. What other items are there on our learning menu? Next, we will tackle the other brain systems that also contribute to learning, look at the phenomenon of forgetting, and say a few words about teachers' roles as 'cognitive enhancers'.

OTHER SYSTEMS INVOLVED IN LEARNING

The reward system's job is to figure out what we need to do to get what we want. In life, we generally want to be given carrots and to avoid sticks. For the brain, the carrot is often delivered in the form of dopamine – that's what we get a little rush of each time someone likes our Instagram post (especially if we weren't expecting it). The modulatory system – that executive – is concerned with turning on and off other systems so that goals can be focused on. It liaises closely with the emotions, listening in to the limbic system and making decisions that integrate how we feel to set goals. This is the system that tunes in to the fact we want to reach for our phone to check Instagram likes to get that little carrot, but suggests that maybe, no, we should finish our homework first.

There are also two other ways that information can be learned. One way is simply by observing other people. As we saw in Chapter 4, many brain networks are built on the need to see, hear and understand other people. We can learn a lot, whether it's practical skills like dance routines on TikTok or socio-emotional skills of how to deal with difficult people – just by watching how other people do it. Finally, the brain has many circuits concerned with using and understanding language, which can be exploited to learn by following instructions.

All of these systems – all the memory systems, the control and reward systems, observation, instructions, and emotions – interact throughout learning. As learning proceeds, shortcuts can be found as patterns are recognised – ah, the 4 times table is just like the 2 times table doubled, poems often use alliteration, essays introduce a question at the start, which gets answered by the end – and, as ever, the brain wants to make this as automatic as possible by making predictions, developing scripts that can run themselves. With all learning, no matter the memory system involved, this automaticity is achieved through practice and repetition – using and reusing new knowledge and newly acquired skills.

WHY DO I FORGET THINGS I WANT TO REMEMBER AND REMEMBER THINGS I WANT TO FORGET?

Well, actually, do you? We're prepared to bet that you actually remember a lot of things you want to remember and forget a lot of things you want to forget. But we know what you mean. It's annoying that you can still remember all the names of the footballers in the Arsenal 1995 squad but can't commit a page of Spanish vocabulary to mind for a test. Just like remembering, forgetting is different in different learning systems. Highly emotional memories of events – those that involve the amygdala – are reluctant to forget what's been learned – things that made us anxious or fearful or exhilarated. Similarly, memories of how to do things – whether it's reading or riding a bike – only form thanks to hours of painstaking practice; they are hard to create and also, thankfully, hard to lose.

By contrast, memories that never really make it past the temporary activations sustained by working memory (as often happens with knowledge that we cram for exams) will be quickly forgotten if the knowledge has never forged meaningful links into long-term memory. In Chapter 5, we also talked about the hippocampus 'filling up' with specific autobiographical memories – typically after about 3 months – so memories have to be moved out to the cortex for the long term. And even long-term memories stored in the cortex depend on being used; over time, knowledge that isn't used will blur and fade until the memories disappear – though repeating particular learning experiences can help to preserve them, and relearning is always faster than initial learning.

There are many pathways to forgetting. In the coming chapter, we will be talking about the many strategies for the classroom that can help minimise the leakage.

TEACHERS ARE BRAIN CHANGERS

If you hear the phrase 'cognitive enhancement', do you think of a gloomy sci-fi film with rows of children sitting trussed up in metallic brain hats talking robotically? Or do you think of a teacher? Because cognitive enhancement is what teachers get paid to do. Their day job is to change students' brains.[6] In fact, if Ms Goodwinch comes home *not* having changed her students' brains, she's had a bad day at work. Another whole book could (and should!) be written about teachers' brains. For now, we just have Box 6.1 Teachers' brains.

BOX 6.1   TEACHERS' BRAINS

Educational neuroscience has focused on the brains of learners. But given the key role of teachers (there are strong links between teacher quality and educational outcomes), should we be thinking

---

6   One recent analysis found that for each additional year a child spends in school, their IQ increases by between 1 and 5 IQ points. The effects persisted across the life span and were present on all broad categories of cognitive ability, leading the authors to comment that 'education appears to be the most consistent, robust, and durable method yet to be identified for raising intelligence' (Ritchie & Tucker-Drob, 2018).

more about *teachers'* brains? What is useful for teachers to know about *all* the brains in their classrooms?

Positive emotions of a teacher are certainly a valuable learning resource. The social nature of brains means we feed off and mirror the emotions and behaviours of others. Enthusiasm and passion are contagious! If you, the teacher, are genuinely enthusiastic about your subject, then conveying that to your students is one of the most valuable things you can do for their motivation – and effective learning. In essence, you are conveying the message, 'Feel how I feel.' Helping teachers maintain enthusiasm for their teaching and their subject areas has great potential value for the whole class.

A recent study (Yeager et al., 2022) examined whether the effectiveness of a growth mindset intervention in maths would be influenced by the mindset of the students' different teachers. Previous research had suggested that the context of support for mindset approaches was a key determinant in their success. The researchers found that, while maths grades were improved for students in classrooms with teachers with a growth mindset, similar gains were not seen in students whose teachers had a more fixed mindset – this group fared no better than controls. The study illustrates just one facet of the complexity of real-world classroom interventions.

Other social and emotional skills of teachers – theory of mind, empathy, managing social relationships, good communication – play a significant role in the classroom too. Teachers need to be expert at gathering clues about misunderstandings and gaps in knowledge, making a diagnosis based on a student's particular mistakes or omissions. They need to do this with 25 or 30 students each presenting with different behavioural clues. And they need to do it while trying to optimise their own emotional state from moment to moment (staying calm and being encouraging, inhibiting signs of frustration, managing others' behaviour). Understanding the importance of emotions and social dimensions of learning is likely to benefit teachers not just in terms of understanding their students better, but also understanding themselves.

Implementing even apparently straightforward practices such as a daily review of learning to strengthen recall and retrieval can be enhanced by understanding how engagement and knowledge building work. Teachers need to notice and remember the knowledge states of different students to provide an appropriate level of scaffolding for each learner. They might consider different environments which might help engage students and minimise anxiety caused, for example, by being called upon publicly to answer questions. They might even consider broader factors such as the role of sleep in consolidating learning – to suggest that a review in the morning of the previous day's learning might be more effective than a similar review at the end of the day.

There are two linked aspects here. One is really to do with teacher training: what are the ideas from neuroscience that are helpful to teachers to better understand and potentially improve their teaching? The other is a proposal: to broaden the remit of educational neuroscience to take teachers' brains and their welfare into account. To ensure effective learning for their students, we should consider teachers' social and emotional needs, make opportunities for their creativity and innovation and develop additional tools to promote teachers' motivation and engagement.

In Chapter 7, we will focus on techniques that teachers can use in the classroom which exploit the principles we've outlined for the brain's learning priorities. Many of these tools will be familiar. In fact, many of the recommendations of educational neuroscience at this early stage of its journey will be based on tweaking and refining things which we already know work. For example, the idea that 'spaced learning' helps retain information dates back many years. Where educational neuroscience can add value is in knowing *how* and *why* something works and so informing the detail of how to make it most effective, given the brain's learning systems.[7]

For spaced learning, how spaced should learning intervals be? How many times should material be revisited? What are the ideal timings of each learning episode? And so on. There is a parallel here with evidence-based medicine. We have known for hundreds

7   Other sorts of questions educational neuroscience wants to help teachers with are: What are the key features of each technique and what can be varied to fit with your specific students and the specific content? How much would you expect a technique to work the same for every child, versus working better for some than others? How could you tell who it will work for? Or when best to use it? All such questions are addressed by a deeper understanding of the mechanism, of how learning works.

of years that chewing the bark of the cinchona tree keeps malaria at bay. But modern medicine has taken this ancient knowledge and fleshed it out – so we now know that it is because it contains quinine, which we can extract (no more nasty bark) and we can specify the dosage, timing and duration of quinine intake most likely to be effective. The goal of educational neuroscience is to save school children from having to chew the bark!

Even when there is research still to be done – and there is plenty that's needed – using a scientific perspective can allow us to make best guesses at effective approaches, based on what we know about how things work. As the field develops, it is imperative that the detailed research into how to maximise the effectiveness of different approaches is conducted with researchers and teachers working together. Classrooms are incredibly complex environments. In scientific parlance, we would say they are full of variables – the physical setting, other learners, the culture of the school, the wider culture beyond the school gates, and, of course, the teachers themselves. Deciphering cause and effect and designing appropriate interventions will rely on collaborations if we hope to devise interventions based on the twin pillars of scientific rigour and classroom legitimacy. Even then, the delivery of teaching will often remain an art, but one powered by the knowledge of science.

FLY ME TO THE MOON

INTRODUCTION

In this chapter, we will give brief descriptions of effective strategies and an explanation of why they work. This book is not a teacher's guide and there is not space to go into all the detail – and teachers have infinitely more expertise when it comes to the detailed planning of lessons. In the Resources section, we have made suggestions for where to go if you would like to pursue these ideas in more depth. We would particularly recommend the 'Practitioner's corner' sections of Sousa's (2011) book, *How the Brain Learns* and the '50 practical applications' in Tokuhama-Espinosa's (2014) book, *Making Classrooms Better*. Our aim here, in the context of building an evidence-based approach to what works in the classroom, is to give a sense, based on some practical pointers, about where we are on that journey and a broad framework to understand why these techniques are successful.

We will not be talking about particular educational systems or specific ways of approaching education. There are many other books which address that. We do not specifically endorse any regime of education and the approaches we outline below apply equally to many different educational environments – different ages of learners, different subjects, different agendas.[1]

---

1   We have drawn on the work of many others in these examples. As well as those mentioned, some of the more important are: Cepeda et al. (2006), Fields (2005), Karpicke and Grimaldi (2012), Kelley and Whatson (2013), Smolen et al. (2016), Yan et al. (2020),; and reports by the Education Endowment Foundation (n.d.).

DOI: 10.4324/9781003185642-7

Broadly, we will describe approaches based on the pyramid of priorities that we have followed throughout this book. These are summarised as:

- *Sensorimotor*: Embody learning, deal with distractions, harness attention, be explicit about where to focus, use concrete examples to help build abstract ideas.
- *Emotions*: Harness motivation, make emotional connections, feedback, reward, strategise to encourage active learning, promote self-efficacy, avoid negative and distracting emotions.
- *Social*: Observe others, teach others (teaching = learning), learn from other people's mistakes and viewpoints, create error-tolerant environments.
- *Strengthen memory*: Use multiple pathways (say it and show it, use case studies and analogies), work with existing knowledge, elaborate, retrieve, test, space out and interleave learning.

CONCRETE EXAMPLES

The brain's sensorimotor systems are foundational to learning. Using specific, grounded examples to help buttress abstract thinking exploits this strength. The result is better learning, as memories are built on more solid and robust foundations. Concrete examples are often used with younger children as they learn about abstract concepts – pizza slices to show fractions or the use of Montessori materials, which are excellent in this regard – but concrete examples can benefit learners of all ages. What 'concrete' means is similarly broad. It could be as simple as the teacher using hand gestures to illustrate the movement of the hands on a clock face. It could be a learning tool produced by students, such as a model of the solar system. Or it could be highly complex – a whole-class enactment of market trading, complete with objects being bought and sold with ersatz money – to embed economic principles, such as how supply and demand affect price. Illustrations, songs, poems, physical gestures can all be used to help link abstract ideas to the realm of the sensorimotor system.

ANALOGIES AND METAPHORS

Most abstract concepts are built on sensorimotor analogies (Lakoff & Johnson, 2003)[2] and teachers often (both spontaneously and deliberately) use sensory and motor analogies and metaphors to teach them. The key challenge is to ensure that the student takes the correct features from the analogical domain and ignores the irrelevant ones. For example, think of the analogy that electrical current is like the flow of water through a pipe. This depends on specific mappings: water pressure being seen as voltage, and the width of the pipe as resistance. But other mappings need to be avoided: the student shouldn't take from the analogy that electricity is wet.

One way around possible mapping problems is to supercharge the approach by using *multiple* analogies. With more than one analogy to draw on, students can triangulate to find the key aspects of the abstract concept and discard irrelevant sensorimotor features. With the electricity example, an additional analogy might involve seeing the system as a big loop of rope, with a person (acting as a battery) pulling the loop through their hands. Resistance is represented by someone holding onto the rope, making it harder to pull. Putting together the water-pipe and rope-pull helps clarify the relevant concepts while avoiding distractions such as the materials (water, rope) themselves.[3] All analogies have limitations: for alternating current, the water flow/rope has to be thought of changing direction many times a second, which is not easily imaginable.

The message here is that analogies and metaphors can be of great help in the classroom since they represent a way of making ideas more concrete without the need for the actual concrete materials. But great care and explicit direction are needed to ensure that students are making the right – and only the right – connections.[4]

2   Also see Lakoff and Núñez (2000). Their book's poetic subtitle is 'How the embodied mind brings mathematics into being'.

3   For more science analogies, check out https://www.furryelephant.com/content/electricity/teaching-learning/electric-circuit-analogies/.

4   Watch a recent CEN seminar on 'The cognitive science of teaching and learning with analogies', available at: http://www.educationalneuroscience.org.uk/events/seminars/.

MULTIMEDIA LEARNING (INCLUDING DUAL CODING)

Working memory has two main pathways: one to process visual/spatial information and one to process sound, usually verbal information. Learning can be strengthened by information being given in *both* modalities, since this offers two opportunities for encoding. Visual information can come in many forms – graphs, cartoons, mind maps, infographics – the important thing is that it contains relevant information and isn't just there to add colour without purpose. Visual information could mean pictures given to students to aid learning or pictures created by students to help them understand and make learning more meaningful to them. And verbal information does not only mean the teacher speaking – it can be our own internal voice as we read our notes, or our peers, as we work with them on a project. Once materials have been produced, it's a good idea also to practise retrieving the information in both forms to strengthen memory.

BOX 7.1   WHAT WORKS IN MY CLASSROOM?

There is a pyramid of ideal educational neuroscience research. Its solid base is a scientific approach to the classroom, with teachers carrying out their own small studies to test new or current practice. Promising approaches can then be tried on a larger scale with greater rigour, building up gradually as evidence of benefit accumulates. So how do you go about assessing what is going on in your own classroom? How can you tell whether your new way of teaching phonics or fractions or fission is better than the old one? Here are a few key principles:

- *Decide on your research question.* What are you doing? What are you expecting the result to be? How do you plan to measure it?
- *Comparison.* You should use your new technique on some students and not on others and see which group improves most. You might want to compare with another new approach (maybe a fellow teacher has a different promising idea) or with existing practice – or both.
- *Control group.* This is a special kind of comparison which allows for the fact that just being in a study can influence results (e.g., children are excited, you are excited). You want it to work for

the reason you think – it's your new innovation. So your control group should be doing something as similar as possible but without the new innovation.

- *Randomisation*. To avoid other factors muddying your results, you should allocate students randomly to different groups. Randomisation can be as simple as drawing names out of a hat to say who goes in which group.
- *Data collection*. You need to decide in advance what you are going to measure (a test on fractions, a reading comprehension with set follow-up questions). You should give it to the children in all the groups before you try your new innovation (to get a 'baseline' measure, this is called a pre-test) and then again afterwards (a post-test). Even if both groups improve, this allows you to see who improves most.
- *Be objective and be blind if you can*. When we want things to work, we can inadvertently look for confirmation that it has done so. It is important to be as objective as you can. Ideally, you won't know which child was in which group (that's what 'being blind' means) though this is sometimes logistically difficult.
- *Analyse the data*. Depending on the data you have collected, you will need some simple techniques like comparing average scores in different groups, to see how the students have performed. You might also want to look at whether the new approach has had different effects on different children in any systematic way (e.g., girls vs boys). Who does your new innovation work best for?
- *Think ethics*. Are there any risks in what you are planning to do? Is it fair? Could there be any unintended consequences?

For more information and resources, have a look at the Centre for Educational Neuroscience website: 'What works in my classroom', available at: www.educationalneuroscience.org.uk.

PAYING ATTENTION

The brain is constantly paying attention. The task for the classroom is to make sure it is to the right thing. Learning happens through both focused and peripheral perception and it is often difficult for students to know where the priorities are. A simple but important principle is to tell them! If learning objectives are clearly outlined and the path to achieving them is well described, that's a good start. When new content or activities are described, highlighting the key sensory and motor features is important. In addition, planning activities which grab attention are a good way to set things off on the right track. The brain likes novelty, so anything new – in the classroom set-up, the materials, the manner of the teacher, a surprise visitor – will help alert students. Humour is also a very helpful tool for grabbing attention. Remember that attention is built on sensorimotor systems – classroom attention is just an evolution of what our ancestors did: take notice of all the sensory input in order to generate the right action in response. It is not surprising, given the dynamic environment of a classroom, that help is needed to point it in the right direction.

AVOIDING DISTRACTIONS

Good attention is made more difficult by confusion about what to focus on. Classrooms are full of distractions, both external – other students, noises, displays, technology – and internal distractions – hunger, discomfort, mind wandering. Interventions to reduce distractions are likely to help attention. Reducing internal distraction is a lot to do with motivation and engagement, which we'll come to shortly. But one way to improve mind wandering is to name it. Teaching students about their own mind wandering, helping them to identify when it might happen or is happening, and teaching them how to refocus are a simple way to help. The idea of helping students understand the control they have over their thinking is a potentially valuable and underexploited part of metacognition, which we'll talk about more at the end of the chapter.

Ways to reduce external distractions, based on our 'best bets' (there is a lack of robust research), are to try to keep classrooms quiet if focused attention is needed (collaborative group work might be an exception) and to keep visual displays to a minimum unless they are relevant and will be referred to in what is being learned. Alternatively, displays can be kept just for the back of the class, away from where students are facing. In terms of technology, there is strong evidence that the use of technology which is non-academic (things like texting, using social media) is associated with worse learning and not only for the user but also for those around them. This points to avoiding technology in the classroom. However, technology covers a huge amount more than social media – and the pandemic years have shown just how crucial technology is when schools cannot operate as normal. So while avoiding the sort of distractions of social media apps is a good idea, other uses of specific technologies in the classroom should each be judged on their own merits, considering both costs and benefits.

MOTIVATION

Motivation is a crucial determinant of the amount of attention we are prepared to give. Harnessing motivation for learning can have a powerful force multiplier effect – an engaged student will be more actively involved in learning, seek out their own examples, elaborate naturally, share learning with others, and so on. Teachers, of course, know this. But how to achieve it? Much of what good teachers practise here is likely in line with the brain's preferred diet. Activities, social engagement, collaboration, finding relevance and meaning are all good; turgid textbook information delivered by a teacher going through the motions – not so much. More broadly, teachers determine the class environment – emotionally as well as literally – and can lay the groundwork that supports learning. Students come with different levels of motivation – as with cognitive ability, individual differences in motivation are partly heritable and partly environmental. Teachers cannot necessarily remove all of these differences. But each individual can improve from where they are and teachers can help with that. The message here then is less one of new insights, and more a corroboration of existing best practice, much of which is designed to enhance motivation, whose importance it is hard to overstate.

CHALLENGE NOT THREAT

Our brains respond to all kinds of threats. Even though we sometimes present this instinct in evolutionary terms, with exotic examples like poisonous snakes, in the classroom, the same instinct is at work. Here it might warn of much more subtle threats – a teacher whose responses are unpredictable or whose tone of voice carries a sense of danger can be perceived as threatening. The risk of embarrassment in front of peers can also be perceived as threatening. And perception is everything. It doesn't matter whether the fear is founded or not, since the perception of it is usually enough to elicit the sort of stress response which is not conducive to learning. By contrast, a teacher who encourages student's sense of their own belief that they have the potential to learn and improve can have a huge effect on motivation and engagement. A motivated learner will respond to high expectations because they will see them as achievable. In a nutshell, learning is enhanced by a sense of challenge and reduced by a sense of threat.

CONNECT EMOTIONALLY

If emotional connections can be made with what is being learned, it will be remembered better, since emotional memories are stronger. Connecting information being learned to things that are meaningful for students is not always easy (since it can be highly individual) but will pay dividends. Teaching students about their emotional responses to learning can also help make them more aware of how to take advantage of them. Greater awareness by teachers of how students perceive them (the teacher) and their learning is also helpful because perception, as with perceived threats, is what matters. Incorporating positive emotional messages into teaching and embodying emotional control even in challenging classroom encounters are likely to benefit everyone in the classroom.

A key point to reinforce here is that emotions are not separable from thinking. Emotions are a critical component of the brain's systems for pattern detection and decision-making. Learning does not happen without emotion. In fact, *learning* new information is more influenced by the emotions than *retrieving* information; anything that can be done in the classroom to create positive feelings about learning will pay dividends in better retention.

TEACHER FEEDBACK

Feedback plays a very important role in learning. We all know from our own lives how highly emotional an experience getting feedback from others can be. Whether these emotions are positive or negative, their potency means that memories of feedback times are likely to be strong, so it is important to make them count. The aim of constructive feedback is to give guidance without causing negative side effects. Teachers should also be mindful of the timing of feedback to maximise the chances of positive outcomes. The best feedback is authentic, specific, and based on evidence, ideally using illustrative examples from the student's work to minimise the risk of misunderstanding. It should focus less on outcomes (whether something was right or wrong) and more on the processes involved. This idea is at the heart of the 'growth mindset' approach which emphasises the work done rather than the result obtained. Feedback should be seen as a learning tool in itself; if it happens at a point when the student herself or himself has realised there is a gap in understanding, and feedback can help understand and fill that gap, it is likely to constitute a potent learning moment.

ENHANCE SELF-EFFICACY

Students' beliefs about their ability to learn profoundly affect their actual ability to do so. This is a blessing and a curse: the virtuous circle of teaching a confident learner is matched by its counterpart, the vicious circle of teaching someone who does not believe in their own ability. One of the most important jobs for a teacher is to encourage and imbue a sense of confidence in students. They can do this through the classroom climate (their own manner being nurturing and encouraging, the culture being one in which students celebrate each other's successes, collaborative rather than competitive), through not judging or labelling students, and more directly in their feedback (see above). Particularly for students with low self-belief, teachers should try to find small examples of success as often as possible, to help students gradually reframe their belief in themselves as capable learners. Short, low stakes quizzes to check learning in small units and which are pitched at a level where most will succeed can be helpful in this regard.

CELEBRATE ERRORS

It is a rare student who naturally celebrates making a mistake. But mistakes present great learning opportunities, so it is important to try and bring students round to that idea. As we have seen, the brain has developed to really pay attention when its predictions are wrong – when it makes an error. It is what stimulates it to review the evidence so that the prediction will be better next time around. Students who are open to error (as well as being open to uncertainty and new experiences generally) will learn faster, because they are able to exploit this machinery: the more errors, the more opportunities for the brain to correct itself. So there is little more illogical in the classroom than creating a punitive environment for mistakes; such an environment turns its back on one of the best learning opportunities. Fear of being laughed at by teachers or peers for having a go and getting something wrong runs counter to learning, especially since we can also learn a huge amount from the mistakes of others. Creating an environment which is open to hearing ideas of all kinds, perhaps especially those which don't match our own, is helpful for learning. Teachers themselves can be very important models in celebrating rather than shying away from their own mistakes. Although we have discouraged over-adorning the walls of classrooms, we might make an exception for a poster that says, 'Mistakes are learning opportunities.'

RETRIEVAL PRACTICE

Retrieval practice involves recalling information from memory with the help of prompts. The approach is based on the idea that memories and the pathways that connect them can vary in strength. Strengthening memory means both embedding it more deeply in existing knowledge and reinforcing a frontal control structure that says, 'In a context with these cues, access these memories.' The aim then is two-fold: (1) to recall specific memories more readily; and (2) to broaden the cues for retrieval so that they are wider than just the specific conditions of learning, so that the relevant knowledge can be applied to new problems.

As we have seen, the act of recreating memories by recalling them itself strengthens and reinforces that knowledge, since the memory must be rebuilt each time. This helps to make the memory more accessible and the access to it more durable. The rebuilding of memory can be prompted by simple quizzes, typically carried out frequently and with low stakes, to help students see what knowledge they have retained and can retrieve. Since retrieval quizzes themselves build learning, they can act both as a learning and an assessment tool.

The theory is very well established but there are still questions regarding the detail, for example, the extent to which there should be variation in the recalled content or whether keeping things very similar to the original learning is better. It's also important to emphasise that retrieval is not the same as restudying: just re-reading or reviewing material is not usually effective, since it does not require the active recreation of knowledge from memory. In addition, care must be taken to check that students are not retrieving the wrong information (for example, an earlier misconception they might have had) since the act of retrieval will then serve to reinforce incorrect knowledge. It is important for students and teachers to check that wrong information is not being recalled and reinforced – even formative assessments need to be marked. There are also many ways that students can prompt their own retrieval, such as with the help of flash cards or mind maps.

SPACED LEARNING

Students nearly always need to engage with new information several times because content systems in the cortex change slowly. If teachers give students the opportunity to reinforce concepts, memory pathways will be strengthened through the long-term potentiation of neurons (that is, neurons becoming more likely to fire when they receive a stimulus). Concept formation, as we have seen, relies on experiencing enough learning opportunities to overlay them and draw out commonalities.

There is strong evidence that spacing out episodes of learning will make for better retention than delivering the same amount of learning in a block. For spacing to be effective, the learner must actively be processing and focusing on the learning, not just blindly repeating it – since its effectiveness relies on the repeated retrieval and rehearsal of knowledge to alter neural connections. Spacing within lessons, for example, in ten-minute chunks with a different activity in between, as well as spacing between lessons, when sleep comes between times, which also promotes further consolidation of learning, have both been shown to be beneficial. One of the early educational neuroscience projects, funded by the Education Endowment Foundation and the Wellcome Trust, was called 'Spaced learning' and was all about refining the detail of the spaced approach. See Box 7.2 Case study: spaced learning.

BOX 7.2 CASE STUDY: SPACED LEARNING

The spaced learning project was an intervention designed and led by teachers in the Hallam Teaching School Alliance in the UK and funded by the Educational Endowment Fund (EEF) and the Wellcome Trust. The intervention tested knowledge retrieval in science using a spaced learning approach: content is taught intensively multiple times, with breaks in between. Here, it involved three repeats over an hour – three sets of 10 minutes of science teaching, interspersed with 10 minutes of a physical activity, such as juggling or origami. This same schedule was repeated for an hour each day on three consecutive days. The intervention was delivered within the normal hour-long science lesson.

Behind the intervention was the idea that, while teachers knew of the general principles that make spaced learning effective (see more on this on p. 143), they were interested in the fine tuning: How spaced? Spaced with what? Repeated how often? The study design also exploited the benefits of sleep and of interleaving. The intervention began with piloting on a limited science curriculum before being developed into a large-scale randomised controlled trial involving 125 schools, which would use the high stakes of participants' GCSE science results as outcome measures. Based on the pilot results, there is the expectation that this could prove a low-cost, high-impact approach but unfortunately, at the time of writing, the results are not yet in. The pandemic delayed the final evaluation (which, in line with EEF guidelines, is carried out by a third-party evaluation team, separate from those who ran the intervention – such due diligence is time-consuming!). The report is due in 2022/3. Watch this space.

As so often, there is nuance. There is evidence that teaching two very similar *motor* skills (hitting a ball with a tennis racket and hitting a ball with a rounders bat) close together can be detrimental to learning (Sousa, 2011). This is probably because of interference in establishing separate automatic motor programmes. So here the advice would be to avoid teaching such things on the same day, and on teaching the second to explicitly highlight the differences from the first. For the dancers among us, don't mix together learning the tango and learning the foxtrot, your brain will get confused. Learn the tango, then learn the foxtrot afterwards, focusing on what's different between the two dances. This example highlights a principle we have come across several times: different knowledge systems have different preferred diets of experience. Here, the ideal diet of spaced learning for the conceptual knowledge system in the cortex differs from what works best for procedural learning in the motor system.

INTERLEAVING

A similar idea, 'interleaving' describes switching between different types of problem or different ideas within the same lesson or session of study. If, for example, you are studying history topics, one might be about the Cold War, one might be about autocracies and one might be about the causes of the Second World War. Intuitively, it would seem that learning each of these in separate blocks would be most effective, so as not to get confused. In fact, the evidence is that mixing them up results in better long-term learning.

There are a few reasons for this. First, going away from a topic gives the opportunity to forget material; having to retrieve it (that is, using working memory to reactivate it within long-term memory) strengthens it. Second, connections made between topics will help to strengthen the memory of them, since they will embed in more networks, offering more routes for retrieval. Third, there is a well-established effect of 'primacy' and 'recency', which means that we tend to remember things at the start and the end of a teaching block better than the bits in the middle. By having multiple smaller blocks, we are creating more starts and ends.

ELABORATION

Elaboration involves adding detail to knowledge, chiefly by asking questions about it. This helps meaning, which in turn strengthens memory, especially if the elaboration involves actively seeking out connections between different bits of knowledge. Looking for ways that knowledge can be connected to things in your own life, especially things you care about, is a good strategy. Asking yourself what the similarities and differences between pieces of knowledge are is a useful technique which exploits the brain's ability to find and remember patterns. The more diverse connections that knowledge has to other knowledge, the more retrieval opportunities there are open. If students generate their own material to elaborate on things they have learned, the active nature of the generation itself enhances learning, because it is yet another way in which memories are actively reconstructed. Elaborating on them goes a step further in actively reconfiguring them to encompass the elaborations. Elaboration need not be elaborate! It could be as simple as making up a mnemonic to help remember a particular collection of information.

CHUNKING

We saw an example of chunking earlier when we talked about the capacity limits of the information that can be kept active in working memory. Chunking is a sort of trick, which allows more information to be processed by putting more information into fewer categories. As we become fluent at reading, words become chunks; it is a lot easier to process the word 'didactic' than it is to remember the letters 'd, i, d, a, c, t, i, c'. As we gain expertise in an area, we chunk naturally: a student starting to play music will initially see each note individually, but gradually notes will converge in chunks of bars or longer phrases. Experienced chess players will see whole games rather than individual moves. This type of chunking happens after a lot of repeated practice. But chunking can also be deployed strategically. It can be used to create any kind of categories, which then become the new chunks, with additional layers of information buried within them. Creating these sort of taxonomies of knowledge can allow more knowledge to be stored. This might entail students creating lists of 'Similarities and differences' or 'Advantages and disadvantages' as a way of grouping more complex knowledge under a heading. Essentially, chunking makes learning less overwhelming by allowing students to deal with a few key blocks of information rather than many small pieces. Accessing these blocks then enables the student to access the more detailed information within them.

DESIRABLE DIFFICULTIES AND THE ACTIVE LEARNER

Many of the strategies we have described are quite hard. Students are likely by default to retreat to low effort approaches when they are revising; activities such as just reading through, or highlighting, notes of what they have learned is a common example. In a way, the *point* of these alternative methods is the difficulty or, more accurately, the *effort*. It is the cognitive effort, which could be measured in terms of neural activity involved in reconstructing memories, which is doing the work in all these approaches, part of the wider concept of the 'active learner'. Being active takes more effort, it uses more energy, than being passive. How we *experience* effort, or use energy, is hugely variable. We can spend hours running up steps and throwing ourselves around in a waterpark, expending huge amounts of energy that we barely notice, while the energy of walking two extra minutes due to a closed bus stop can feel unbearable. The difference? Motivation. It is at the heart of whether we are prepared to make effort – and raising motivation to supply the requisite mental oomph is a great approach if achievable. When motivation feels out of reach, the best bet is for teachers to be very mindful of the mental effort required by each activity and adjust the dosage, the duration and the timing to keep things manageable.

TEACH IT TO SOMEONE ELSE

Most of us have probably had the experience of explaining something to someone else, and only then realising the gaps in our own understanding. Teaching someone else is one of the most active forms of active learning since knowledge must not only be retrieved but also articulated and communicated effectively. In addition, teaching reciprocally compels learners to see their knowledge and understanding through the eyes of someone else, which can help elaborate and reinforce understanding. It requires assumptions, questions, and uncertainties to be articulated, which can lead to higher-order thinking. In the language of the brain, the encoded knowledge is being asked to broaden and flex to drive a wide range of motor responses: sentence generation, gestures, drawings, all of which rely on a mental model of what the social partner understands – which means it must become more flexible and robust.

Work in small groups, such as pairs, is often helpful in reducing the anxiety sometimes caused by speaking and performing in public. Clearly care is needed to make pairings which work for both halves of the partnership, as well as to ensure that what is being shared is accurate. Attention is needed to keep on topic and ensure that the social priority of the brain does not get in the way; it will not be helpful if a student is so preoccupied about how they are coming across that the content itself becomes secondary. If practical constraints limit the feasibility of group work, even the thought experiment of *imagining* explaining something to someone else can be a helpful learning tool. Sometimes this is thanks to the imagining itself highlighting gaps in knowledge which can then be deliberately filled. At other times, the simple act of imagining is sufficient to trigger a kind of internal rearrangement of our knowledge which allows us, by means we do not fully understand, to fill in knowledge gaps by ourselves (Lombrozo, 2017).

BOX 7.3   TEN PRINCIPLES OF TEACHING

1   Plan for repetition, within and between lessons, terms, and years.
2   Feedback often, with kindness and specifics.
3   Train students to think about their thinking – make thinking visible.
4   Use testing to improve learning (as well as to measure).
5   Encourage students to work in groups with shared learning goals.
6   Take time to work out what motivates each child.
7   Treat physical activity seriously (while making it fun).
8   Teach the same thing in different ways.
9   Welcome in the physical world, with cues and examples.
10   Create an environment where errors can be celebrated.

TRANSFER

Transfer describes the ability to take learning from one situation and apply it in another. Given how the brain works, this is a difficult task, since without explicit instruction otherwise, knowledge lies in silos. Nonetheless, transfer remains something of a holy grail for learning. The idea that there might exist some superpower at the top of the learning pyramid which, if we train, cascades down to many other levels has proved a stubborn one. Article after article suggest such possibility: 'How learning to play a musical instrument can boost your IQ'.[5] 'Chess returns to the timetable: Schools reintroduce game in attempt to improve children's brainpower',[6] despite years of evidence that such a magic bullet does not exist. Remember, as we have seen, the only bona fide method we currently know for improving general intelligence in children is education itself.

Some degree of transfer does happen automatically. If we know how to drive a car and we then play Super Mario Kart, we can transfer a great deal of knowledge – of how to steer, accelerate, break, avoid obstacles – from one environment to the other (probably not a great idea to test transfer the other way). If we know the word for love in French is 'amour', when we are in Italy and hear the word 'amore', we see the connection. We spot patterns that we recognise from one situation in another. When knowledge is reactivated via working memory, associated knowledge can also become active in long-term memory that connects to, or is similar to, the new information. As well as offering up connection points and overlaps, past knowledge is essentially recycled into the current learning and can help give it meaning.

TRANSFER DISAPPOINTMENTS

Over the years, there have been many targets of hope for transfer 'miracles'. The tale of transfer disappointment dates back over a century (Thorndike & Woodworth, 1901). Recently, *working memory* has been set up as the miracle emissary. You won't be needing a spoiler alert …
The problem here stems from working memory being wrongly conceived. As we saw in Chapter 6, it was (and often still is) conceived of as a general-purpose mechanism which any kind of content can be moved 'into' or 'out of' as if it were a bucket. This created wrong expectations about what training might achieve – training would enlarge the bucket! Or training would put the bucket on wheels to pick things up and drop them off anywhere! *If* such a general purpose processing mechanism existed (as it does in the digital computer where this metaphor for working memory originated), this expectation might

5   *Daily Mail*, 27 October 2009.
6   *Daily Mail*, 12 November 2012.

have been realised. The reason it hasn't is because the whole concept is wrong: working memory is not a general-purpose bucket that can be filled and emptied. Rather, it is the ability to reactivate, maintain and manipulate the contents of long-term memory systems. If a task which involves working memory improves, what has improved is the brain's ability to use its frontal cortex to reactivate, maintain activation of, and manipulate a particular set of content in those meaning systems – visual systems, spatial systems, auditory systems. This doesn't *generally* improve the ability of frontal cortex to do the reactivating, maintaining, manipulating job, and it doesn't improve the ability to carry out these operations in *different* meaning systems or with *alternative* content. It just improves the ability to carry out that particular task.

Neuroscience gives us an accurate portrayal of how working memory works, based on biological constraints (content is stuck in the structure of the system), which means we can make more accurate (and less miraculous) predictions about the likely effects of training.

Working memory certainly plays a very important role in thinking and learning and there is strong evidence of association between working memory performance and achievements in arithmetic, reading and overall educational attainment. Working memory ability also improves steadily throughout the school years, which suggests it might be more amenable to intervention than if it were already fully developed when children start school. So there has, and continues to be, much interest, both in schools and from commercial companies, in training it; many of the 'brain training' games that are available are targeted at improving working memory. But to reiterate: although working memory *can* be improved with training, training effects are typically specific, short-term and do not generalise (Melby-Lervåg & Hulme, 2013). This is fine if there is interest in improving a specific skill but disappointing if the hope was to train one thing and see cascading improvements elsewhere.

It is not all gloom and doom, however. Building on our understanding of the brain does give us an idea for an approach that might be more successful. It is the idea that we need to *train students in transfer*. This means we recognise that transfer will not happen by some magical secret process but may happen with the help of explicit instruction. We approach transfer not as some mystical superpower but as a skill that can be trained. The skills involve teaching students to approach a new situation with the idea of searching through their previous knowledge, skills and strategies, to see what might be relevant. It is teaching students to think about their thinking and learn about how they learn. It's more meta than Zuckerberg. It's called metacognition.[7]

METACOGNITION

In earlier chapters, we have seen that each of our brains is constructed on the basis of our unique individual experiences in the world. Any single experience only produces a partial representation, specific to its particular context. A partial representation means a set of neurons activated by that particular context – it contains the relevant knowledge (relevant in the sense of what the teacher wants to teach), as well as all the neural, physical, and social context in which the knowledge was formed. This knowledge is spread throughout the brain, not in a storage box, but widely distributed. If and when it is reactivated, it is as an approximation of the original, not a perfect facsimile. It is likely to be a better approximation if it is elicited in a similar context than a totally dissimilar one. In fact, it is often hard to activate knowledge in a different context. Partial representations do not easily transfer. To transfer knowledge to a new context – key to meaningful learning – means the brain being given lots of chances, multiple exposure to enough partially overlapping representations. Revisiting knowledge in different contexts and repeated practice accessing it are key. Teaching which explicitly highlights the commonalities – the overlaps, the bit we are trying to learn – is the final piece in the puzzle (Hobbolog, 2016b). It's about equipping the brain to recognise the cues in the new situation that will prompt the retrieval of relevant knowledge.

Teaching for transfer can mean many things. It might mean teaching how past learning can help current learning. An example might be an explicit task such as asking students to recall what they learnt about the causes of the First World War to see if those can help explain the causes of the Second World War. It might mean teaching how current learning can help future learning. For example, teaching students

7   The other alternative to bring about generalised improvement is to improve the overall functioning of the brain. Give it more energy, better nutrients, lower blood cortisol by reducing stress, strip out metabolic waste with a good night's sleep. This is the brain health approach to far transfer.

how to read a graph (highlighting the key sensory and motor features: the lines of the different axes, or the different types of graphs, such as scatterplots, bar charts, line graphs) means that when they encounter graphs in other subjects, they will be able to see the similarities. More complex teaching for transfer might involve using metaphors and analogies to draw out links between separate pieces of knowledge. Good teachers already do many of these sorts of things, making links and connections to add meaning to new learning situations. Teachers are the most crucial agents of transfer.

The idea of metacognition takes these a step further, formalising the process of thinking about thinking and learning. Metacognition involves monitoring the thought processes involved when you are learning, identifying when you have hit a problem and knowing how to change tack. An example might be in a task that involves thinking of all the animals you know beginning with the letter 'T'. You might start off by just letting ideas come in, then when those run out, switch to a deliberate strategy, such as creating categories to focus the search: animals that live in the sea, pets, animals you find in zoos, and so on. Metacognition is a key skill for learning at all ages, because it involves the construction of a set of personalised steps, adapted to fit our own thinking processes, that we can follow, i.e., self-regulated learning (Figure 7.1). The first steps in implementing metacognitive approaches

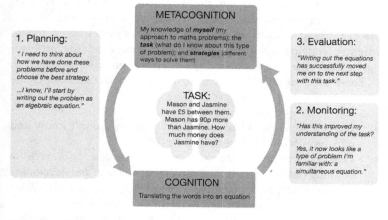

Figure 7.1 The metacognition cycle
Source: Education Endowment Foundation (2018).

are to focus students not on the *endpoint* but on the *process* of getting there. We are less interested in right or wrong answers and more interested in the mechanics. To work well, metacognitive approaches need to encourage introspection – looking at oneself and one's thinking almost as if from the outside. It also relies on teacher feedback. Stimulating metacognition enhances our own knowledge about our thinking and, with practice, improves the monitoring of the thinking process itself. It can apply to all the many aspects of the thinking and learning process – social, emotional and physical factors as well as cognitive ones.

Keeping a 'thinking journal' is one easy way to start with metacognitive behaviours. For students, simply noting times when they have become aware of confusion or uncertainty about what action to take can be helpful, particularly if it is followed up with writing about what happened next – how did they deal with the situation? Over time, this process log can become a useful guide to strategies and approaches to help students take more responsibility for their own learning. Debriefing by teachers can help students become aware of strategies that might be applied in other situations, and those which might be less helpful.

We would emphasise that this process is most effective when it is most inclusive of what constitutes 'thinking processes'. We are not talking solely about 'cold thinking' but the feelings and emotional responses to different stages of the work. Metacognition is as much about identifying 'At this point, I felt really unmotivated because the task ahead seemed so great' as 'At this point I asked myself whether drawing a picture to help me understand the problem might help': the emotional and the cognitive go hand-in-hand.

There are many ways to start developing metacognition. Some common ones are:

- Being able to say what you know, what you don't know and what you would like to know.
- Deliberate planning: this can include practical tasks such as working out how much time something will take and developing rehearsed, reflective cognitive approaches such as asking, 'What strategy have I used before that might be helpful here?'
- Taking time and knowing what to do with it. Using strategies to break down problems into recognisable steps.

- Developing vocabulary around thinking. Modelling is important here so that students can understand what is meant by 'thinking processes'.

Metacognitive skills can be developed at a very young age; 3-year-olds show metacognitive abilities when they are solving problems (Whitebread et al., 2007). Developing these skills at a young age has benefits not only for the student but for the teacher, since making the thinking process explicit makes it easier to spot where problems are occurring. Metacognition makes thinking visible.[8]

The nature of thinking, and metacognitive thinking, changes as children get older. For children younger than about 6, simple tools might help them understand and develop their own emotional self-regulation: a traffic light system where green (go) means you are feeling happy, calm and ready to learn; amber (pause) means you are feeling bored or frustrated, and red (stop) means you are feeling angry or upset, can be a first step in helping children to identify and act on how they are feeling. Children can match their feeling with a signal which points to remedial actions they could try; for example, children identifying themselves in the red zone might identify the action, 'Take 10 slow breaths' or 'Ask to take a break'.

Children in later primary years can be taught more sophisticated strategies linked to particular content or situations. At this age, they are likely to differ greatly in how well developed their executive control skills are which allow them to deploy strategies in the moment; many are still likely to need scaffolding with that. Repeated reflective questions can be a useful touchpoint at the start of and throughout a new piece of learning. This might involve questions about the task (Is this task too challenging? What is hard about it? Are there easier parts? Where is the best place to start?), about themselves (Am I motivated to stick with this when it's tricky? What can I do to keep myself focused?) and about strategies (What can I try if I get stuck? Are my notes helping me understand or do I need something else? Do I need to ask the teacher for help?).

---

8 *Making Thinking Visible* by Ritchart, Church and Morrison (2011) has helpful advice on how to develop 'thinking routines'.

By adolescence, language knowledge and executive function skills are well developed and metacognition can focus on specific items on the syllabus, with study skills classes to target transfer, application of knowledge and skills to new situations, problem-solving, and self-evaluation. At this age, group work and metacognition can be very productive companions. Learning about how others approach their thinking can be helpful in expanding individual repertoires. Practising the art of making thinking explicit by doing it out loud in group work helps to create a culture in which thinking about thinking becomes the norm. It is also likely to be a useful approach for the staff room.

BOX 7.4 INDIVIDUAL DIFFERENCES AND PERSONALISED LEARNING

This book focuses on how brains work in general, for all of us. But of course we are all different. Each brain is built by interaction with its specific environment (from the level of genes and the environment of the womb, through to the level of culture) so everyone's experiences – and everyone's brains – are unique. This presents a massive challenge to educators. And while teachers are acutely aware of their students' differences, it is practically difficult to avoid a 'one-size-fits-all' approach in the classroom. This is not ideal. To give a simple example, we know memory retrieval rates vary. So when teachers give a short amount of time (usually what is practical in a lesson) for students to retrieve some knowledge, this won't be long enough for some students; slower retrievers will miss out on the opportunity to reconstruct and consolidate that learning. The teacher can increase wait time to help slower retrievers, but this might not be the best use of time for the fast retrievers. There is no perfect answer for everyone.

At the heart of *personalised learning* is the idea that teaching should stem from understanding the specific skills, knowledge, strengths and weaknesses of the individual learner. Achieving it would likely improve not just academic outcomes but also individual well-being. Over the coming years, as educational neuroscience focuses on trying to improve personalised learning, its important contribution is to base personalisation on understanding how learning works in the brain. Teachers will know from experience that some students seem to be 'naturally' good at grasping concepts and generalising; those students can then speed through material, for example, by being given problems which allow them to apply concepts to new situations. Other students need much greater repetition of specific concrete examples to understand concepts and clear guidance about how to transfer their understanding to other contexts. The job of educational neuroscience in the coming years is to understand these sorts of differences mechanistically – what are the brain-level differences in approach? – and from this to propose optimal diets of experience to teach different students new knowledge or skills. Sometimes, children who appear to have equivalent problems – in reading or maths, say – have very different underlying cognitive difficulties; one child's underlying problem might be weak working memory, while another might have difficulty with phonological processing. Educational neuroscience can help inform the development of personalised learning tools which tackle underlying difficulties and not just their behavioural manifestation (Holmes et al., 2020).

Technology is often proposed as the key to personalised learning solutions. First, because while teachers can and do monitor student progress, AI solutions are much more powerful at assessing progress digitally; they don't tire of analysing data, can crunch huge numbers in no time and the resulting information can subtly tailor the best subsequent learning to each individual's needs. Second, the COVID pandemic accelerated moves to digital learning, and, third, the best technology for personalising education probably already exists elsewhere – in the games industry, for example. It is only a matter of time before all this is brought together in an economically viable, socially acceptable way.

In Chapter 8, we will move from these general approaches which apply across the curriculum to look at some specific subject areas, seen through our educational neuroscience lens.

COVERING THE SYLLABUS

INTRODUCTION

In this chapter, we move away from topic-general skills that influence learning across subject areas, such as cognitive control and emotion regulation, and instead look at some of the topic-specific skills that apply to literacy, mathematics, arts and science. We reinforce the idea that the brain does not have domain-general components that process any kind of information but rather has content-specific systems, and circuits dedicated to controlling them. We discuss the core abilities that appear to underlie skill in specific areas, such as phonological awareness in reading and number sense in mathematics. Such abilities may be barriers to learning when they are slow developing, or alternatively may present opportunities to accelerate learning. We go on to look at some approaches common to teaching the arts and the sciences which can be beneficial to both.

We have talked about the brain in terms of its general operation — pattern recognition, memory systems, integrated emotions, attention — but in education, we have to learn specific things — how to read, how to do sums, how to dissect anything from a Maya Angelou poem to a frog. We are so accustomed to reading and writing and to the conventions of maths, it is easy to forget just how many different processes have to be efficiently brought to bear to perform these activities without even thinking. In the arts and sciences, additional processes which support creative and critical thinking and manage higher-level concepts, get in on the act. In the next sections, we will break down some of those to better

DOI: 10.4324/9781003185642-8

understand the core of complex activities, point to places of possible weakness and suggest means of amelioration.

LITERACY

Wouldn't it be handy if the brain had a nice neat separable 'reading module'? Sadly, it doesn't. In fact, to read this sentence, you are using and coordinating the activity of at least 16 different neural networks (Tokuhama–Espinosa, 2014). Achieving fluency in reading takes thousands of hours of practice. Teaching a young child to read effortlessly is one of the hardest things we can ask them to do.

If we think of the typical new reader, a child of 4 or 5, they have just spent several years learning to speak. They've got pretty good at it and probably quite enjoy being able to communicate. We are now going to throw at them the idea that there is a whole other world of communication – that those words they've become competent at saying out loud can also be expressed in terms of different marks of ink on a page. In English, we have 26 of these different marks (52 if you count both capitals and lower case) and we call them the letters of the alphabet (we also divide them into vowels and consonants, but that's not down to their shape that's down to the sounds they make; bear with us here). And then, of course, there are punctuation marks, which relate in some mysterious way to the rules of grammar and also whether you are saying something, or shouting it, or asking it as a question.

We are going to intrude on the child's painstakingly constructed spoken language system to attach a whole new system based on recognising these written letters and trying to match up the shapes they make to the sounds in the words that they can speak. It's actually much worse than that, because, at least for English, the matching is really imperfect – some of the letters make more than one sound (think of the 'o' in 'lots', in 'women', in 'onus' or in 'goo'), especially when they're joined to other letters, and some of the sounds can be made with different letters (the sound 'ay' can be made with 'ai', as in 'wait', with 'ay' as in 'say', with 'ey' as in 'hey', or even with 'eigh' as in 'weigh').

There is the additional challenge that the written letters can be represented in a huge variety of ways (Figure 8.1).

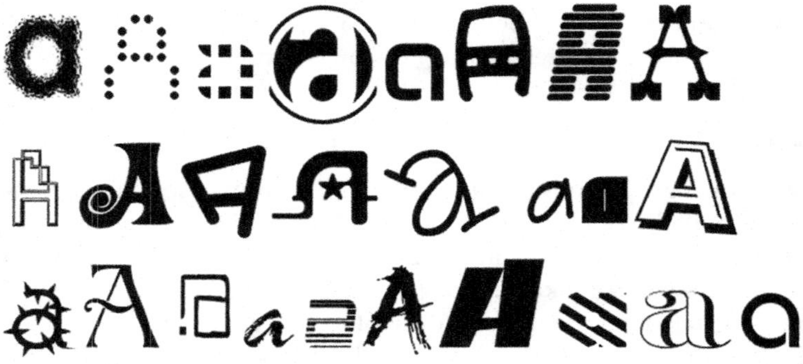

Figure 8.1 When is an A not an A?

As if that weren't enough, certain letters do not obey important rules that the child's brain has taken the preceding years to painstakingly learn. For example, the principle of 'rotational invariance' describes the fact that the visual system has evolved a procedure for recognising objects no matter which way up they are. The toddler learns to recognise that their teddy bear is still their teddy bear when it has fallen off the bed onto its head. Their sippy cup is the same sippy cup whether they are seeing it from above or from the side or from underneath. It is an important aspect of development, achieved by having many object detectors all over the retina, which store all the different views of that object and categorise them as the same thing.

Then they enter school and start learning to read and they meet the letters b and d and p and q or the numbers 6 and 9. To the visual system of the child, these are all just a long line with a round bit stuck on, because the system being used to interpret them is designed to see them in that way. It's not just that children confuse the letters or muddle them up, it is that they are having to learn the rules of a whole new system of visualisation, *unlearning* what they know about objects. But *only for reading!* No wonder it can take years to overcome the brain's natural preference and see these letters as distinct, as well as mastering all the various forms they come in.

This brings us to an important principle that arises from how the brain developed. In many aspects of learning, we take a system (the visual system in the case of reading) which evolved to allow it to develop a particular adaptive purpose in response to a particular environment and we train it to do something else, in a different environment, at a different time.[1] To get a sense of the principle, let's take an analogy: if you have a screwdriver but you need a trowel, you can go ahead and use your screwdriver to dig up some earth but it is certainly not the perfect tool for the job; it will take a lot more effort and involve a good deal more mess to dig your hole. This is the idea that if you are stretching something to work in a different environment it will face challenges and might have to reshape to fit that environment (attaching additional pieces of metal to the head of the screwdriver to widen it could help dig a better hole). The analogy gives the gist of the idea of repurposing; however, it breaks down in the sense that evolution does not directly shape high-level cognitive outcomes, instead evolution gives the brain the plasticity, the flexibility, to develop these outcomes when it finds itself in a typical environment.

When our Sumerian ancestors started carving into clay tablets 5000 or so years ago, they set in train a process by which we all began to recycle our brain parts (the term 'neuronal recycling' has been used to describe this idea).[2] We took parts evolved to visually analyse faces or footprints and instead started using them to recognise letters and words. Thanks to brain imaging, we now understand a great deal about the mechanism of reading. And thanks to some Ronseal (does what it says on the tin) naming, we know that the key recycled area is the Visual Word Form Area (VWFA). This part of the brain, which is activated when we see a written word, is the key visual contributor to reading in all cultures that have been studied. So reading is not a 'natural' activity. It has not been around for long enough to be encoded in our genes.

---

1   The phrasing here is deliberately slightly tortuous: we are trying to avoid language such as 'the brain evolved to …' because it gives the sense that evolution knows where it is going, when of course it doesn't. The point here is a subtle one: the struggle with reading is not that we're repurposing a system constructed by evolution to do visual processing of objects (evolution doesn't care what we use it for, only that we have babies); it's because the typical developmental process operated for 4–5 years to use the brain's plasticity to do visual object recognition – so reading involves having to undo learning that has already occurred. Indirectly, the problem comes from evolution selecting a brain whose key characteristic is its flexibility or what we refer to as brain plasticity.

2   See Dehaene (2010).

Unlike spoken communication, which has evolved and developed because of its role in survival, reading and writing are much newer.

The process of reading (greatly simplified) goes something like this. Step one, decode the visual input into shapes. Step two, learn the relationship between these shapes and the speech sounds that make up our spoken words (the reading system is, in a sense, parasitic on the oral language system). Bring to mind the spoken word that the string of symbols corresponds to. And then retrieve the meaning, just as you would if someone said the word to you. Except the brain is cunning. Over time it starts to learn direct links from the visual symbols to the meanings, so it doesn't have to go through the long-winded letters-to-sounds translation process. It's complicated to learn but allows for much greater speed and is a very handy back-up when the mapping of letters to sounds is particularly opaque, such as in 'aisle' or 'yacht' – don't bother to translate these, just head straight over to meaning. The process involves the visual system, the auditory system, and language areas to contribute information from stored word knowledge and the frontal cortex to bring it all together and add meaning.

In reality, this is an incredibly sophisticated and finely tuned feedback system rather than a simple linear process. When we read, our eyes skip along the line of text, alighting to read a couple of words at a time before the next jump.[3] If a word does not make sense, or doesn't fit with the context, the uncertainty will prompt the visual system to re-read it. Our eyes somehow never land on a word like 'and' or 'the' at the centre of our visual field. They settle instead on rich content words, the nouns and the verbs. How do they know to do this before they have had a chance to read what's there? To avoid something they haven't even seen yet?! Well, when we are expert readers, as we read the words our eyes have alighted on, out of the corner of our eye, we see a blurry preview of the words coming up next – at least whether they are short or long. And our brain can deliberately programme the next jump to land on a big word and ignore the little ones, which are more likely to be grammatical or function words. The expert brain has learnt the most efficient way to

3   These jumps of the eyes are called 'saccades'. If you want to see how jumpy our eyes are, watch someone's eyes closely as they read or, better still, as they look out of the window of a moving train.

process the text, by focusing on the most meaningful words for understanding the content of the sentence. And it all happens in parallel (several word sounds being processed at once) and in a fraction of a second. High fives all round for our brains.

In terms of how fluent reading develops over time, we can break the process down into a series of stages:

1   *Metalinguistic awareness.* This refers to the ability to break language down into its constituent parts and manipulate them. It has three components. Phonological awareness describes the awareness of the sounds that make up our language (for example, what does 'Paris' sound like if you take off the 'P'?). Morphological awareness is the awareness of the structural similarities and regularities in the words of the language (for example, in English, plurals usually end in 's', the suffix 'un' changes a word's meaning to its opposite). Orthographical awareness is awareness of the visual nature of written words, such as seeing regular word forms and spelling patterns (for example, spotting words that are likely to rhyme, such as 'blind' and 'kind' and 'find').

2   *Alphabetic principle*: mapping oral (spoken) language onto writing systems. This means learning to recognise that written symbols represent speech sounds.

3   *Practice for pattern recognition.* Practising complex pattern recognition takes up a big part of the development of literacy. It requires students to make very fine discriminations between very specific visual stimuli which takes a long time and involves two distinct but related processes: (a) making fine discriminations between sometimes very similar patterns (see Figure 8.2); and (b) grouping subtly different forms together (letters or characters written in different ways). Although what we see on the outside, when a student is learning to read, is explicit teaching and deliberate effort on the part of the learner, it is the exposure to a huge amount of data – that is, to many words, in many contexts – that is the key to the statistical learning that is going on beneath the surface. The more data it has access to, the faster the brain will become at recognising the patterns. *And still more practice for fluency.* This is to emphasise the amount of time and practice involved to

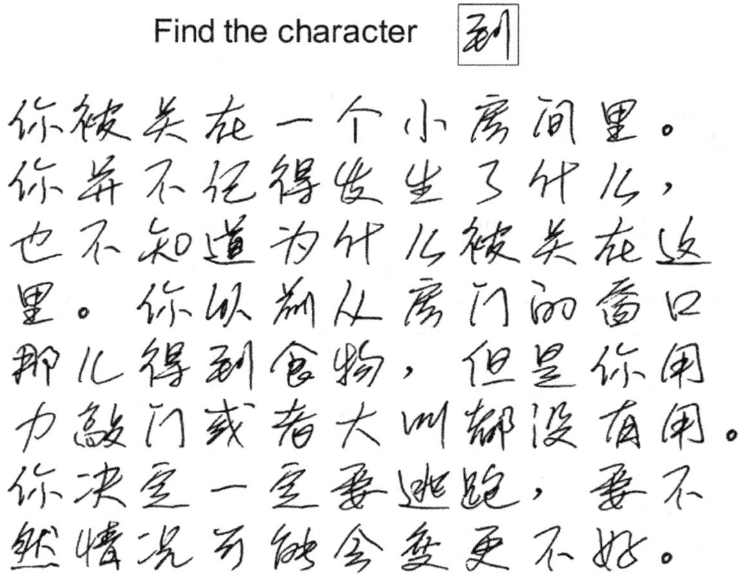

Find the character 到

你被关在一个小房间里。
你并不记得发生了什么，
也不知道为什么被关在这
里。你以前从房门的窗口
那儿得到食物，但是你用
力敲门或者大叫都没有用。
你决定一定要逃跑，要不
然情况可能会变更不好。

Figure 8.2 Complex pattern recognition, such as the fine discrimination needed to make out specific characters, has to happen incredibly fast for reading to become fluent

achieve reading rates of roughly 60–100 words per minute, which is an estimate of what constitutes fluent reading. After the heavy lifting of earlier stages has been done, there is still the need for a huge amount of practice to speed the process up sufficiently to lower the effort (that is, how much the front of the brain has to work to provide focused attention), to allow concentration on meaning, and even, in an ideal world, make it enjoyable.

Teaching literacy offers something of a showcase of many general best-practice principles of educational neuroscience. For example, metalinguistic awareness is all about bedding in the sensory and motor foundations of reading, in the context of active, explicit learning and with concrete examples. Practice perfects the instant pattern recognition needed to turn slow, effortful procedures into fast, automatic ones. And given the large amount of practice required, motivation is key; content selection (ideally by the child themselves) is hugely important to ensure that the child stays motivated enough by the material they are reading to put in the necessary effort. This is not the time to push unwanted content.

Reading is such a complex ability that there are many ways that it can go wrong. One of the best-known difficulties is developmental dyslexia, in which children with adequate intelligence, typical senses, and sufficient environmental stimulation, have difficulty learning to read. Neuroimaging has helped to identify the brain regions typically affected and the main causes of difficulties. These include specific phonological deficits, phonological memory deficits (that is, difficulties associated with employing working memory to keep the representations of phonemes active), differences in the speeds of auditory and visual processing (meaning, for example, that the visual system is moving more quickly than the auditory system can keep up with). Patterns of brain activity could be a useful predictor of children who might need intervention and potentially could offer earlier prognosis than behavioural markers; some researchers are even exploring whether the way in which infant brains respond to auditory signals (measured by electrical activity on the scalp) may be a useful way to predict the risk of later literacy difficulties (Benasich et al., 2014). New 'neuro-interventions', such as transcranial electrical stimulation (tES), are also being trialled to see if stimulating the VWFA to boost its plasticity can address deficits, and neuro-diagnostic tools which allow the structure and function of auditory cortex to be mapped also offer potential new routes for intervention and earlier diagnosis.

NUMERACY

Maths, like reading, is a culturally, rather than genetically, acquired skill that has to be explicitly taught. In the same way that reading instruction exploits structures in the brain evolved to support the development of language, maths exploits other brain structures which appear to underlie the understanding of quantity. And, again, just as with reading, learning maths means hijacking systems which have not developed in a way optimised for this purpose. Additional neural circuits need to be persuaded, by explicit instruction, to join in, in another example of neuronal recycling. Maths provides a sort of test case for how the brain reorganises itself to respond to the demands of education. This active construction of maths skills and knowledge largely takes place in the classroom.

Although we think of maths as a single thing, it is actually a very diverse set of things for the brain. A neuroimaging study which looked at people's brains when they were completing sequential subtraction (100 minus 7, minus 7, minus 7, etc.) identified ten distinct brain areas that were involved (Dehaene, 2011). Even the simplest maths operation is widely distributed in the brain, requiring coordination of many different areas; number representation itself involves bringing together circuits involved in magnitude sense with visual and verbal representations.

Think of the many operations involved in even a simple piece of arithmetic, such as $2 + 3 = ?$ Answering it involves decoding the number symbols 2 and 3, decoding the rule symbols ('+' and '='), extracting from memory the rules of addition and 'is equal to' they represent and keeping active in working memory the words 'two' and 'three' in order to apply the addition rule. Seeing the pattern might be sufficient to allow you to retrieve the correct answer. But that's not enough! The teacher wants your brain to 'understand' addition. That means adding in a lot of extra facts – that $2 + 3$ is the same as $3 + 2$, that $2 + 3$ is 'close to 6' but not 'about 10'. Getting to this thing called understanding will involve practice using different strategies (counting up, counting on), extracting knowledge of numerical magnitude, cross-referencing results with learned principles (e.g., addition produces numbers of larger magnitude). All this means embroiling extra circuits, building linkages to language systems and practice with different content and in different contexts to achieve the ultimate 'abstract' concept.

To succeed with this in a classroom setting additionally means being able to read, staying focused enough to attend to the problem in hand and inhibiting visual, auditory, or internal distractions. It might also mean overcoming feelings of anxiety, low self-belief, or fear of getting the answer wrong. When we do maths, many brain areas come together to integrate all these different systems and procedures. There are many ways that maths learning can go awry (OECD, 2007).

Just as the visual word form area is a key brain hub for literacy, the (unfortunately less catchily named) inferior parietal sulcus is the home of number sense. It is part of the parietal lobe of the brain, which, you might remember from Chapter 2, is involved in body sense – processing spatial information linking the body with sensory information. Mathematical competence is grounded in children's active experience of the world and the use of their bodies, particularly their fingers. It should come as little surprise by now that sensorimotor learning comes first. With maths, fingers are our handiest early tools for representing the numbers 1 to 10. Finger sense (also known as 'finger gnosis') describes the ability to identify and distinguish between our individual fingers; neuroimaging studies have shown that early experiences using our fingers to represent number (such as when we count on our fingers or point to our 'fourth' finger) create a lasting neural impression (Soylu et al., 2017). Transcranial magnetic stimulation studies show that changing the levels of activity in the inferior parietal sulcus affects both number processing and finger sense.

This area is consistently activated in number tasks and appears to be active even in non-human primates. One highly trained chimp, Sheba, demonstrated an ability to perform simple arithmetic using both concrete and symbolic representations of number; first, by collecting groups of oranges hidden around a maze (two first, then three somewhere else) and selecting the answer '5' from a selection of digits; then performing this same feat with Arabic numerals instead of oranges (Boysen & Capaldi, 2014). Imaging studies similarly found that Sheba was activating the parietal lobe.

This evolutionary appreciation of number has some important attributes. The first is that most people can enumerate sets of up to three or four objects without counting them, a process known as 'subitising'. We see a small number of items and the brain just knows how many there are. This is likely an object tracking ability, part of our visual attention system, which operates before we get into counting. A second is the 'distance effect', the fact that reaction times for distinguishing the bigger of two sets increases as the distance between the number in each set decreases (that is, it is easier to distinguish 10 and 20 than 10 and 11). The rate of change of this effect (as difference in relative set sizes goes up or down) is remarkably consistent in humans and monkeys, again suggesting a common underlying neural process.[4] The third and most fascinating fact is that numbers in our brains seem to be represented on a sort of mental number line. The line, at least for English-speakers, is oriented from left to right with smaller numbers on the left and larger numbers on the right. Children get used to the spatial arrangement when they encounter numbers in a line, with numbers increasing from left to right − and this pattern becomes imprinted on their brains. This means that when people in test settings are asked about the relative size of two numbers presented on a computer screen, they will respond more quickly with the *right* hand to answers about which number is larger, and with the *left* hand when asked which is smaller. This finding, fascinatingly, is reversed in Arabic-speakers, who use a right–left written system. The number line allows for efficient and automatic processing of quantities, since it means the brain can automatically 'see' where numbers are in relation to one another. And it underlies what we think of as number sense, a necessary foundation for mastering maths with greater degrees of complexity. Perhaps the key insight here is that the brain is not only treating numbers as a sequence of symbols (though it can and does do that when the counting sequence is retrieved) but also as a display existing in physical space to which actions can be notionally directed.

Symbolic number processing, such as the ability to link symbols with quantities, in the early years is a reliable measure of how well children will likely get on with maths. In addition, phonological processing ability and phonological working memory are critical components. Reading and arithmetic share overlapping brain networks, since phonological processing is a key ingredient in the retrieval of number facts and phonological working memory is needed to retain interim calculation facts, rules, and strategies for long enough to be useful. In fact, since phonological working memory has been so regularly associated with maths ability, there have been many interventions focused on improving it to improve maths overall. As

---

4 This likely comes down to broadly tuned quantity 'detectors'; for similar numbers (10 and 11), their detectors both get activated, and it takes a moment to see which detector is more active to trigger a decision on which is bigger, while, for far apart numbers (10 and 20), the activity of their detectors is easy to distinguish.

we have already seen, hopes for far transfer, that is the transfer of learning in one context to another, quite dissimilar one in such interventions, is usually thwarted; learners will improve on the specific trained phonological working memory task, but generally not beyond.

More promising numeracy interventions provide good illustrations of some educational neuroscience principles in action. For example, playing linear number board games such as 'Snakes and ladders' gives multiple cues about number order and magnitude: the higher the number in a square, the greater the physical movement the child has to make to reach it, the more number names she has spoken and heard, the greater the distance she has travelled and the longer the amount of time that has passed since the game began. These sorts of games are a living embodiment of the mental number line. They require manipulation of physical concrete objects, they involve speaking aloud, movement, seeing and hearing numbers represented in different ways simultaneously. Even more important, they are social and they are fun. And evidence suggests they work (Siegler & Ramani, 2009).

The development of more difficult arithmetic skills involves a gradual change in the predominance of different strategies with experience. More than many subjects, maths development requires earlier stages to be thoroughly learnt and embedded, since subsequent learning is built on these foundations. Although this is true for all learning, poor foundations can be particularly damaging for further maths learning, and even a possible cause of particular anxiety about maths.

A lot of arithmetic development is about doing the necessary practice to make laborious processes automatic. Early on, efficiency improves as counting strategies move, with sufficient rehearsal, from the concrete (e.g., fingers) to the abstract in the head. Automaticity becomes the norm as, with repetition, number facts (number bonds, times tables, rules such as addition being reversible: $2 + 9 = 9 + 2$, etc.) are stored in long-term memory. Retrieval from memory has the advantages of being more reliable (as long it has been stored correctly), faster and of putting less demand on the requirement of frontal cortex to keep temporary representations active. It also means that harder sums can be done without needing to keep the whole process in the head; for example, if I ask you the answer to 4 x 2, you can probably just say it automatically – it is there as a memorised fact. It comes out fast and accurate. 4 x 13 might be the same, if you took your times tables that extra step, but more likely it involves a set of procedures – either doubling and redoubling 13 or holding the answer to 4 x 10 in mind while you calculate 4 x 3 to add to it. 4^3 involves an additional step which is the retrieval of what the x^3 operation involves, then deciding on the solving strategy, then proceeding as before. Slower, more laborious, more prone to error.

Dyscalculia is the number equivalent of dyslexia, a developmental difficulty associated with specific maths impairments (Butterworth, 2005). Although still less recognised than dyslexia, between 5 per cent and 7 per cent of children are estimated to be affected by it. It can occur on its own, in children with no problems with general intelligence, but more commonly it is seen alongside dyslexia or ADHD, implying either a wider constellation of affected or detuned brain systems or a common underlying cause. The problem in dyscalculia is that numbers are simply not meaningful; those with the condition typically lack the foundational skills of enumerating, estimating relative magnitudes and of recognising small number groups without counting. As such, it tends to affect arithmetic more than other maths skills (spatial cognition, for example, is often not affected). Searching for the best amelioration of the condition is an active area of educational neuroscience research.

ARTS

In a book like this, we would typically expect to see literacy and numeracy tackled, while the arts are often neglected. Why might this be? Throughout human history, the arts – dance, song, visual arts, drama – have been a part of culture, an essential part of our lives and the stitches of our social fabric. But when it comes to traditional Western education, the arts are often side-lined or forgotten. We would argue, from the position of educational neuroscience and what makes the brain tick, that this is an error. The arts play a key role in development – social, emotional, sensorimotor, and cognitive – and they continue to enrich our experience throughout life. From the point of view of the brain, the arts align with the brain's needs – there is a reason why they have always been a part of human culture. And in the modern world, the 'twenty-first-century skills' deemed critical for students – creativity, collaboration, critical thinking and communication – are all central to teaching and learning in the arts.

For babies, toddlers and young children, we consider it completely natural that they should dance, sing, paint, play, listen to and make up stories. Gradually, as they grow older, these activities which once felt like natural desires, driven by social, emotional, physical and creative needs, start, for many, to ebb away. There is curriculum chauvinism common in educational settings, which has maths, English and science at the top of the hierarchy, humanities in the middle, and the arts at the bottom. It's almost as if they have taken our diagram of 'things the brain really cares about' and put the arrow round the wrong way (Figure 8.3)!

Many specific qualities and practices in the arts are fundamental to brain function. Specialised parts of auditory cortex are responsive just to the tones of music. The acuity of the visual processing system allows artists to see, recreate and reimagine the world in ways tightly tethered to or completely unshackled from the real world. Much of the work of the cerebellum is coordinating precision movements – the pirouettes of a ballerina or the acrobatics of a capoeira performer. Drama relies on interactions between the limbic system and specialised language areas in the cortex to

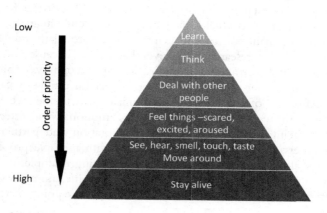

Figure 8.3 The arts go hand in hand with the brain's priorities

convey character with clarity, conviction and emotional richness. An intriguing study gives an illustration of just one unique way in which the arts can push us to deploy sophisticated and unusual mental operations. In an fMRI[5] scanner, actors were asked to respond to questions either as themselves or in character and their brain activity compared in the two situations. Compared to being themselves, being in character produced overall reductions in brain activity, particularly in certain parts of the frontal control areas. Stepping into the shoes of another character involves, literally in a brain sense, a 'loss of self' (Brown et al., 2019). This finding links to another key feature of the arts, which is their social aspect – their ability to allow us to communicate without words, to imagine worlds beyond and better than our own and to help our societies survive and prosper.

There are many creative and critical competencies which are most readily learned through the arts. These include learning to use the imagination as a substrate, being able to adapt and shift practice in response to changing goals, seeing the importance of detail and nuance, all sorts of problem-solving, such as working out how to convey an idea without spoken language, flexibility in working with constraints while also seeing the possibilities of challenging those constraints, working with others, and seeing the world from other people's point of view. And, of course, the arts often use our bodies in new ways and they carry rich emotional components. They make us move and they make us feel.

Some schools take the approach of ringfencing set times for the arts, such as in 'Arts weeks' or 'Music weeks', but integrating the arts into the main curriculum seems to be a particularly powerful approach. Some researchers believe that this is because the arts generate ideal learning conditions and metacognitive abilities which can transfer to other areas (e.g., a 'playful mindset'). Some of the features of arts learning are familiar from themes we have explored throughout this book: being emotionally invested in what is being learned, learning in collaboration and partnership with others, working on specific projects with multiple problems to solve along the way, hands–on learning using multiple, diverse types of input. Parents and teachers often become more involved in arts collaboration projects since they offer up more points of access.

5   Functional magnetic resonance imaging. See Box 1.1 Tools of neuroscience.

This in turn enriches the experience and makes it more authentic. The arts can be of particular benefit in motivating students who struggle to otherwise engage, whether that is because they are generally disaffected with school, or they have neurodevelopmental disabilities or learning styles which mean they are not engaged by traditional teaching methods.

As we will see in the next section, there are many parallels in arts and science learning. In simplest terms, both involve learning the skills needed to make close and detailed observations of things in the world, and the skills to move beyond these to create and experiment. Earlier, we saw the error of seeing the binary of 'cold cognition' being rational, logical and useful while 'emotional cognition' is flighty, impulsive and irrational. In reality, 'rational thinking' *requires* emotional thinking; they are inextricably connected by the notion of value, and the way the brain processes them – and the best decisions are made when both are given appropriate weight. There is a parallel with the arts and sciences: our brains thrive when we combine the best of both.

Recent neuroimaging work has shown some unique features of creative thinking. In particular, creativity involves collaboration between brain networks which normally don't work together. In non-creative thinking, the frontal cortex, where executive control (the modulatory system) resides, turns down or off our internally focused thinking – so that we are not distracted by mind wandering and other streams of internal thought. In creative thinking, these networks instead work together, exploiting those inner thoughts to achieve external goals. For example, improvisational jazz musicians turn down their executive control when they are performing so that they can access those harder-to-reach inner dialogues (Limb & Braun, 2008). The famous jazz saxophonist Charlie Parker was on to this idea of finding a balance between freedom and control when he said, 'You've got to learn your instrument. Then, you practice, practice, practice. And then, when you finally get up there on the bandstand, forget all that and just wail.'

SCIENCE

Science has a reputation for being hard to learn (Millar, 1991). There are a few reasons why. Although students are often interested in the subjects that science addresses (whether those are big issues like climate change or ponderings like why the sky is blue) they often feel that science in lessons does not quite deliver the answers they want. Science can be very abstract, even early on and sometimes it is difficult (or insufficient time is given) to make it more concrete and meaningful with hands-on examples. It can also involve highly effortful reconstruction of meaning, since many things learned in science conflict with everyday life experience (in life, the ball does not just roll off the edge of the football pitch but in science, the world is round). And in the way it is taught, there is sometimes a conflict between an enquiry-led approach where students are encouraged to seek out their own questions and answers, and the transmission of more brittle science knowledge which involves difficult concepts and vocabulary.

Early on in development, concept formation relies heavily on sensory input. A child drops a pebble into a pond and it disappears to the bottom. With repeated exposure to similar scenarios, the child forms an idea of the causal pathway involved and develops a 'sinking schema' which allows her to predict what will happen in future scenarios. This process is facilitated by language labels, but even pre-language, infants are sensitive to these sorts of causal pathways.

As childhood continues, more elaborate concepts develop and these are gradually and increasingly separated from perceptual representations. In other words, perceptual and conceptual systems have different developmental trajectories and can be differently activated in response to the same task – even if this leads to conflicting results. Perceptual systems allow the brain to predict what will happen next, while conceptual systems allow explanation, and the two may be out of step. Causal concepts develop at different rates, depending on the quantity and quality of outside input, which chiefly comes from concepts being explained by someone credible whom the child trusts (a parent, a teacher, an older peer). An important point arising from this is that there can be conflict between earlier, incorrect perceptually based understanding and later, more theoretical, language-based understanding. This knowledge has been used as the basis for a school science intervention geared to improving primary school science outcomes. See Box 1.2 Case study: 'Stop and think'.

The practical implication is that science teaching should build explicit links between perceptual and abstract conceptual understanding.

Learners need to see how things are in the real world, and then be guided with frameworks to help think through the logic of causal pathways, which can then provide a basis for grasping established scientific ideas.

The actual language of science should not be underestimated as a factor in learning (Dockrell et al., 2007). The speed of vocabulary gains in the early years has perhaps led to an assumption that children will also acquire new science terms readily. In fact, it seems that in the early years, the acquisition of science terms can be hesitant, if the words come before schemas have been constructed and if words do not relate to concrete things. This illustrates the complexity of the links between concept formation, perceptual information and language learning. This in turn connects with recommendations in Chapter 7 regarding the use of analogies in science and the importance of grounding abstract concepts in sensorimotor systems, as well as the challenge of ensuring that the student takes the key properties of the analogy and not the unintended ones – this is the challenge of levering blue sky abstract thinking out of the brain's comforting hold on the sensorimotor.

In addition, science learning, like maths, develops and accumulates sequentially. We have to learn things in the right order and learning relies heavily on building on the formulas, theories and concepts that have been previously learned. The consequences of missing lessons can be significant since foundational concepts might be missed. Also, if early knowledge is not thoroughly embedded, problems can accumulate quickly.

There has been a good deal of interest in the benefits of problem-based learning approaches in science. And although these approaches are by no means new, an educational neuroscience lens can help us understand more about why they work – and in time, adapt them to improve learning outcomes still further. Generally speaking, problem-based learning approaches begin with the teacher presenting a problem. It might be something local: how to make the school plastic-free, something global: how to prevent rain forest destruction or anything in between. The choice of problem is important – it needs to be messy enough to allow multiple solutions, ideally of a changeable nature and with lots of variables. It should not be something that can be solved easily, such as with the application of one specific formula and clearly it needs to be a problem with many possible good responses as opposed to a single, obviously best one.

As the problem is tackled, the role the students take is very active – it is up to them to unpick and unravel it, while teachers are there as cognitive (e.g., addressing issues relating to problem content or construction) or metacognitive (e.g., asking questions about strategic approach) guides. Students work in groups, sharing information, ideas, and approaches – but each learner constructs their own knowledge individually in a way that is personal to them. Discussions, provocations and challenge – in an environment which explicitly encourages constructive dissent – serve to expose problems, test thinking and lead to collaborative revision. Ideally, assessment accompanies the process and not just the product.

From all that we have seen so far, we can identify many possible theoretical reasons why such approaches should work. Motivation is front and centre, learning is active and what is being learned is (assuming problems have been well chosen) relevant to the real world. Anxiety can be reduced by the fact that work is shared with a group, lessening individual exposure, and given the right environmental conditions, quieter group members have a better chance of active involvement than in a full class setting. The format promotes higher-order thinking and more self-efficacy, since the focus is not 'What answer does the teacher want me to find?' but 'How can we, as a group, set our own judgement criteria for what tackles the problem effectively?' Metacognition is encouraged (and can be explicitly so), as students generate strategies for defining the scope of the problem, researching, and gathering information, analysing data, building and testing hypotheses and experiments to test them, comparing, and critiquing different approaches and sharing methods and conclusions. An interesting research finding is that, in acquiring the skill to form hypotheses, it seems to be crucial to hear other people talk about what is going on – even if what they are saying is wrong. The experience appears to train the brain that other views are possible and encourages the practice of adopting them before perhaps dismissing them because they don't fit the evidence. This means both language and the social group context play an important role in acquiring the apparently dry scientific skill of forming and testing a hypothesis (Howe et al., 2000).

The Education Endowment Foundation toolkit suggests collaborative approaches are a low-cost, effective way of improving outcomes, with particularly high impacts in science. Students engaged in collaborative learning interventions make an average of 10 months additional progress over the course of an academic year (compared to 5 for similar approaches in maths and 3 for literacy). The approach is successful in both primary and secondary settings, with recommended group sizes of 3–5 students, ideally working towards a joint group outcome.

Some challenges of the approach come from difficulty finding good problem examples, since as well as all the problem criteria stated above, problems need to be commonly understood by all students. In science, it could be counterproductive to work on problem-solving in an area where some students have not fully understood its foundational principles. The key with teaching, then, is to strike the right balance between discovery learning and explicit instruction.

The example of collaborative approaches is a good illustration of aligning the brain's priorities: its social priority now working in the service of the conceptual. Science learning can also be aligned through exploiting sensorimotor systems. One recent research project tested whether enacting physical processes could aid learning; researchers used a model involving bicycle wheels which spun independently on a single axle (and which students could handle and manipulate) to allow students to learn about angular momentum by physically *feeling* it (Kontra et al., 2015). The researchers found that these short but meaningful physical experiences, which activated sensorimotor systems involved in similar actions in the past, significantly improved test scores for students in the bicycle wheel group compared to control groups. This sort of embodied cognition[6] approach offers up many possibilities, particularly in the areas of engineering, physics and chemistry.

In Chapter 9, we will return to the overall goals of educational neuroscience. What are some of the key social, political and ethical issues which might arise as this fledgling interdisciplinary field begins to stretch its wings? In the meantime, we will leave you with ten key takeaways for teachers about how the brain works.

---

6   For an introduction to the ideas of embodied, or 'grounded' cognition, see Barsalou (2008).

BOX 8.1 TEN KEY TAKEAWAYS ABOUT HOW THE BRAIN WORKS

1   The brain is always paying attention.
2   The brain likes to make things automatic.
3   The brain can't help making predictions about what is going to happen.
4   Emotions are not an 'optional extra'. Physical and mental health, emotions and cognition: these are not separable.
5   Counting on your fingers is a good example of how the brain bolsters abstract learning with concrete examples. It's not cheating.
6   The brain builds itself and changes throughout life. Different parts change at different speeds at different ages.
7   The brain undergoes enormous repurposing during adolescence which triggers a burst of socio-emotional learning.
8   Practice makes permanent – so make sure you're practising the right thing.
9   Learning is a lifelong activity for the brain. The more you do, the more effective it is.

THE WHOLE-SYSTEM PERSPECTIVE

INTRODUCTION

Educational neuroscience is not all about brains. Any attempt to improve learning will be doomed if it fails to consider the multiple factors, operating at many levels, which affect learning outcomes (see Figure 9.1). Beyond the brain, there are individual-level factors: physical health, nutrition, sleep, exercise. There are family-level factors; what support and resources do children have at home? Do they have access to technology? Do they live with stress or violence? What is the attitude to learning at home? There are classroom factors: what is the skill of the teacher? Is the classroom environment conducive to learning? What is air quality like? Are teaching materials sufficient? How do school policies and priorities impact individual learning? And, finally, there are the broader cultural factors which affect the whole educational enterprise; what is valued in the education system? Is education free and available to all? What resources are available for spending? Do governments and societies care about equality? What is the cultural consensus on diversity and inclusion? In this final chapter, we situate learning in its broadest context. This perspective makes clear that the educational neuroscience endeavour only makes sense if it is truly, passionately, steadfastly interdisciplinary.

'BRAIN SCAN TO LESSON PLAN'

Despite the catchy phrase, a simple model in which the findings of neuroscience research are simply handed over to teachers to put

DOI: 10.4324/9781003185642-9

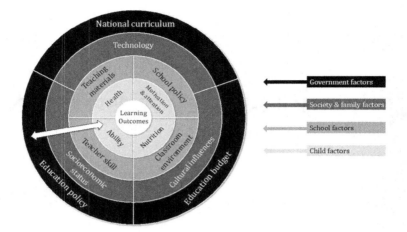

Figure 9.1 Local and distant factors that influence learning outcomes and the interactive relationship between the individual and the environment. The white arrow reflects the two-way influence between layers.
Source: Thomas et al. (2019).

into action in the classroom has never been the expectation. Most neuroscientists have no classroom knowledge, their research is typically focused on scientific questions rather than pedagogical ones and research has generally not been informed at any stage by what teachers or schools or students want and need. That is not how the story of educational neuroscience unfolds. Rather, the field requires that educators and scientists (and not just neuroscientists, but also cognitive, social and developmental psychologists) work collaboratively. Meaningful dialogue means everyone stepping a little outside of their comfort zone to understand the perspectives of others. There is much that is shared but different terms for similar concepts, different values and professional objectives, different timescales and practical needs can obscure the common ground. As well, there are many points of difference; sometimes, the most pressing scientific questions might not align well with the problems that most vex teachers.

Educational neuroscientists sometimes look to the history of medicine as an inspiration for the move to a more evidence-based approach, but there are enormous differences between comparing the effectiveness of two medical treatments in a set of patients and comparing two classroom interventions. Classrooms are some of the most complex environments that exist. Among 20 to 30 children of differing abilities and temperament, there is the complication that what works well for one child might not work well for another. Teachers also vary hugely and we know that teacher quality is one of the strongest predictors of educational outcomes. Isolating the effects of interventions themselves, when they are delivered by differently skilled teachers in different settings is difficult. Classrooms, schools and geographical regions or areas also vary greatly.

Even an intervention with a very large effect in the controlled setting of a lab has many many stages to pass through before it can even be released 'into the wild', with multiple potential fracture points along the way. For educational neuroscience to progress, it needs to overcome many practical obstacles and work hard to find clarity in complexity by embracing diverse disciplinary perspectives. It needs to develop creative, innovative methodologies which give due weight to both the social and the natural sciences and to allow their contribution to be meaningfully and appropriately brought together. Let us take the example of the UK introduction of a phonics test for 6-year-olds in 2012. Phonics, as we have mentioned, is the ability to 'sound out' a string of written letters. Researchers found that children's ability to read out loud both real words and non-words (made-up words in English that look like real words, e.g., *plave*) was a good predictor of whether children would later struggle with their literacy. A screening test was designed for 6-year-olds. It meant that extra resources could be targeted to children who scored below a threshold to reduce future risk of dyslexia. It addressed the problem that later diagnosis, say, at age 9 or 10, makes remediation harder; the child has already fallen behind and may have experienced damage to their self-esteem.

When this test was released 'into the wild' as a national screening programme, several unforeseen problems arose. First, the teaching unions boycotted the test because they felt formal tests were not appropriate for children of such a young age. Second, schools feared that performance of their children on this test would be used by government to judge the quality of their literacy teaching, so they felt pressure to 'teach to test'. (In fact, research showed differences in children's performance on this test were less to do with quality of teaching than heritability.) In a similar vein, concerned parents, keen to help their children in their first formal test, were tempted to practise reading non-words at home, undermining their role as novel strings of letters. Third, children's test performance was marked by teachers; analysis of the distribution of test scores suggested children scoring close to the pass mark were being 'boosted' over the threshold – there were fewer than expected marks just under the threshold.

In its transition from theory to practice, all these real-world factors impacted on the effectiveness of the test for its intended purpose, despite the great potential of the test to improve children's educational outcomes and support struggling learners. These real-world effects are not 'bugs', but rather features of the complexities of the educational neuroscience system.

THE GOALS OF AN EDUCATION SYSTEM

Societies and governments set the overall goals of the education system. But even once we have decided on an educational approach, how do we ensure it is best delivered to students? Do we want to improve outcomes across the board for all students? Or make sure that no one is left behind, for example, by setting a minimum level that all students must attain? Alternatively, do we focus on excellence and seek to extend and expand learning for those of highest ability? Or is our priority reducing wide gaps in educational attainment, bringing everyone's outcomes closer together? Figure 9.2 illustrates the broad, population-level effects of some of these different approaches.

These are political questions more than scientific ones. It is beyond our scope to answer them. Rather, we mention them to highlight the fact that changes in the classroom need to be considered in this wider context. Decisions for paths taken invariably involve opportunity costs. If, for example, a government sets new attainment requirements for literacy and numeracy for all, that means time in the classroom that is no longer available for teaching arts or sport or humanities. Or it means students spending longer in education to catch up, with opportunity costs for other parts of

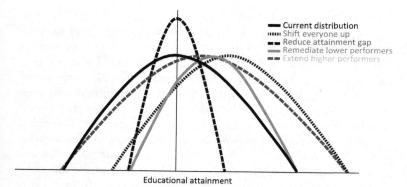

Current distribution
IIIIII Shift everyone up
■ ■ Reduce attainment gap
Remediate lower performers
■ ■ Extend higher performers

Educational attainment

Figure 9.2 Representation of the effect of different educational policies on the overall population distribution of educational attainment

their lives. These might be positive, if those other parts are not enriching, but equally could take away opportunities for students to explore passions and interests.

NEUROETHICS

As educational neuroscience develops, it also needs to consider ethics. Are there research areas that should be prioritised or avoided? How do we decide whether it is acceptable to experiment on children in classrooms, as we inevitably do when we try new educational approaches? What are the additional ethical questions raised by educational neuroscience over the ethics of education generally, given that the goal of *all* education is cognitive enhancement?

As we have discussed, the words *cognitive enhancement* can conjure dystopian images. In reality, though, just drinking coffee or going for a walk to clear the head are types of cognitive enhancement. Teachers' jobs are all about cognitive enhancement; the goal of education is to change brains. But artificial enhancement – boosting the brain with chemicals to alter neural activity or stimulating it electrically to improve certain functions, such as memory – feel like a next step. Early evidence suggests that the appetite for these approaches might depend on what they are being used for. For example, a recent study found people viewed 'neuroscience-derived applications' more favourably if they were being proposed to enhance cognition to an average level for low-achieving students than if they were for high-achieving students to enhance performance further.[1] Another study found that the general public had a greater appetite for pills billed as 'motivational' than for those billed as 'smart', especially if motivation pills were to 'overcome motivational problems'.[2] This suggests that people consider issues of fairness and equality to be an important, if complex, component of decision-making. Sometimes inequality (for instance, unequal provision to help those who are disadvantaged) is the best route to improving equity. There is a related issue in the difference between using these techniques as 'enhancement' versus their use as 'treatment'. Psychostimulants (such as Ritalin[TM]) are already widely used for the treatment of attention deficit disorder (ADD) and are also (illegally) used by healthy students as 'smart pills' to help them study. A recent UK survey involving students at 54 UK universities found that 19 per cent used cognitive-enhancing drugs; their main reasons were to meet coursework demands, improve their focus or maintain wakefulness (McDermott et al., 2021).

Non-invasive brain stimulation usually involves administering a very small electric current via electrodes positioned on the outside of the head. The stimulation changes the resting state of neurons, so that either a greater or a lower input is needed to make them fire. The process is not fully understood but it broadly resembles the potentiation of neurons which takes place during learning. Its effect depends on which part of the cortex is stimulated (that is, where on the head the electrodes are placed) but the idea is that the increased readiness of neurons to fire means that more neurons can play a part in plastic changes to increase future performance.

These techniques are in their infancy. There is little research to date on adults and even less on children. But research, both by commercial companies and academic researchers, is growing fast around the world, so now is the time to think about how we as a society react. What are the risks? If artificial brain stimulation can make positive changes to the brain, it can probably also make negative ones. And there are likely also to be trade-offs.

1 See Schmied et al. (2021).
2 See Faber et al. (2015).

Commonly used psychostimulants (such as those used to treat ADD) have often been reported to cause personality changes (increases in irritability, anxiety, and tearfulness) which sometimes persist even when the medication has stopped. We do not yet fully understand how different individuals are likely to react to interventions though there are a few early clues. A study using stimulation of the prefrontal cortex during a maths training task found that the effect on reaction times differed between those with high and low maths anxiety.[3] There are also questions of access; school results predict life outcomes – so there is the risk that if these techniques are developed commercially, those who can most afford them will benefit most, further increasing already wide educational inequalities.

NEUROMYTHS AND LEARNING ABOUT THE BRAIN

As educational neuroscience matures as a field, it needs to decide on the best approach to addressing 'neuromyths', that is, beliefs about the brain that many people hold but which are not true. On the one hand, these beliefs often reflect an appetite and enthusiasm for neuroscientific evidence, but, on the other, falsehoods about the brain are potentially damaging, for example, teaching narrowly to supposed specific individual 'learning styles' could be detrimental to students. Neuromyths often have their foundation in something scientifically accurate, but they extrapolate from, misinterpret, or misrepresent the science. Sometimes they reflect things we would love to believe. Wouldn't it be wonderful if we only used 10 per cent of our brains or could learn while we sleep – what untapped mental superpowers!

Some of the most common neuromyths are:

- *We only use 10 per cent of our brains*. We actually use all our brain all the time.
- *Intelligence is fixed*. Education is about changing intelligence – none of us would know much if we had never learned it. Although genetics has a role, so does the environment and the two are inextricably interwoven.

3   See Sarkar et al. (2014).

- *Some people are left-brained and some are right-brained.* Yes, the brain has two sides and those sides have some different functions, but we all use both sides to largely the same extent.
- *Boys and girls think differently.* There are some small differences between girls' and boys' brains but there are much greater differences *within* each group than *between* them.
- *There are critical periods for learning.* While there are particularly sensitive periods for some learning (such as the speech sounds of our native language), most skills can be learned at any age.

Teaching should be targeted at a student's preferred learning style. All students benefit from being taught in multiple modalities. Dispelling neuromyths is a matter of promoting good science through good communication. It is not always easy, since, as we've said, many neuromyths have one foot in good science and often represent beliefs at an end of a continuum rather than the wrong side of a line (for example, the difference between 'critical' and 'sensitive' periods is a subtle one). We should also take care not to over-dramatise; currently there is no evidence of a clear link between belief in neuromyths and teacher effectiveness, so it is important not to overstate the dangers and alienate teachers in the process (Horvath et al., 2018).

Evidence should also be gathered to test the theory that improving knowledge about the brain might have a positive impact on teaching and learning. There are some tendrils of related evidence, for example, one study showed that when teenagers are taught about and better understand their brain's plasticity, this benefits their academic achievement as well as their self-concept.[4] Such evidence illustrates a potentially useful broader approach: asking which aspects of knowledge about the brain would be helpful for teachers and learners to empower them to improve their teaching and learning.[5] While the hope is that in the longer term, better knowledge will lead to better practice, we are not there yet. Theoretically sound interventions need to be tested in classrooms to see if they are practical and effective and constitute significant improvement on current practice. Burdening

---

4   See Blackwell et al. (2007).
5   In his book, *The Teacher and the Teenage Brain*, John Coleman takes the view that the role of educational neuroscience is chiefly to inform teachers and learners about how their brains work (Coleman, 2021).

teachers with swathes of additional theoretical knowledge without practical application is potentially frustrating.

Doing this successfully demands an open, collaborative approach. Perhaps teachers have their own set of 'edumyths', beliefs which many (including neuroscientists) might hold but which are not true of education. An open dialogue allows for misconceptions to be aired, dissected, and dispelled, improving understanding and trust on all sides.

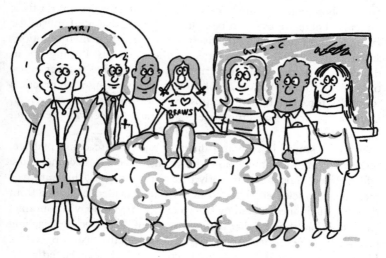

Recently some evidence-based and science of learning views have been introduced into teacher training in the UK. The 2019 Early Career Framework from the UK Department for Education outlines what, on the basis of high-quality evidence, teachers should learn. It includes reference to different types of memory, the role of prior knowledge, how practice and retrieval work and other themes covered in this book. It goes on to give practical guidance about the skills early career teachers need to develop to put that learning into practice. To give an example, the framework points out the distinction between working memory and long-term memory and says: 'Working memory is where information that is being actively processed is held, but its capacity is limited and can be overloaded.' It therefore advises teachers to avoid overloading working memory by 'taking into account pupils' prior knowledge when planning how much new information to introduce, breaking complex material into smaller steps, and reducing distractions that take attention away from what is being taught'. This is hardly revolutionarily new information for teachers. But as our understanding develops, so too will more specific practical advice.

Learning about the brain doesn't just mean understanding *students'* brains. Gaining insights into how their own brains work could also potentially help teachers provide even more effective lessons for their students. There are likely to be many principles that are familiar, for example, most teachers instinctively know that their own emotions about a subject will be transmitted to their students. Putting this in the context of the strong contribution that positive teacher emotions make to the motivation of their students, along with practical strategies for how to convey positive emotions most effectively, could make for more enjoyable – and more effective – learning and teaching.

A recent study[6] looked at a different aspect of teaching practice, motivated by the observation that while teachers become more effective very quickly in the early part of their careers, this improvement tends to level off. The researchers, using evidence gleaned from multiple disciplines, including neuroscience, psychology, economics and education, theorise that the improvement slows because teaching practice becomes more habitual, with unproductive habits baked in. Habits are structured sequences of actions, which are elicited automatically – that is, without thinking – by cues in the environment. Being automatic, they are not sensitive to goals or rewards – or to put it another way, they don't consider their consequences. The danger of habits, which we know the brain loves to form because of the mental energy they save, is that they can automatically continue, even after the benefits they were originally designed for are no longer accrued. When behaviour moves from goal-driven to habit-driven, it is run on different circuits in the brain, so habits work by different rules: changing them involves more than just willpower. It involves employing the same techniques that created the habit in the first place: practice and repetition of the behaviour that's desired in the relevant environmental context.

6   See Hobbiss et al. (2021).

The point here is the brain, as a pattern-recognising automaticity machine, might well carry on using the same automatic programme even when the need for it has moved on. For a teacher, this might mean that simple behaviours adopted early on to establish presence and authority (for example, checking in with students while they are quietly working) become habits, so that silence becomes filled with non-essential chat, which is at best non-productive and at worst could actually interfere with attention and learning. In this respect, educational neuroscience can serve as a lever to encourage teachers' self-reflection about their practice (Howard-Jones et al., 2020).

THEMES FOR THE FUTURE

There are many questions which educational neuroscience has barely begun to wrestle with. How much variation in educational attainment is due to school factors or home ones? What are the most effective approaches to reducing inequalities of educational outcome? Is it most important to work on cross-disciplinary skills (executive functions, engagement, metacognition) or on the foundational skills of literacy, numeracy, science and the arts? How can research be designed so that it meets the strictures of a scientific approach to uncover how and why things work and yet is viable in a range of different classrooms? How can communication between educators, policy-makers and researchers be improved? To what extent should educational neuroscience plough its own furrow or become part of a broader initiative to move to a more evidence-based approach to education?

Over the coming years, there is a lot of work to be done. In the following sections, we consider a few of the areas which are likely to be of particular interest for the field.

COGNITIVE ENHANCEMENT

The allure of new techniques to improve cognition is likely to persist. In recent years, action video games, mindfulness meditation, aerobic exercise, bilingualism and chess have all been considered as potential approaches which might meet the aspiration of achieving widely transferable benefits. Although the goal of far transfer remains something of a mirage, many of these approaches have shown more local benefits: improved attention control of visual processing through playing first-person shooter action video games, improved health and better executive function through certain kinds of aerobic exercise, improved emotional regulation through mindfulness training. On the other hand, some approaches which seemed theoretically promising (playing chess, musical training, increased quantity of sleep) have not withstood real-world scientific scrutiny of their benefits – beyond of course, the obvious joys of playing chess, or music or, indeed, of a good night's sleep.

PERSONALISED LEARNING

Given all we have said about how each individual builds their own brain, how learning is predicated on prior knowledge and so on, it follows that there is great interest in how to personalise learning, that is, to tailor learning to the needs of each individual student. This raises many practical, ethical and pedagogical questions. To personalise learning, we have the potential to draw on a great deal of data – not just demographic and behavioural data but potentially also genetic and neuroscientific data. Are we as a society ready to consider the implications of generating genetic information about a child's educational potential? Even if we are, how can data be safely collected, stored and shared with appropriate stakeholders? At a practical level, how could these sorts of data be effectively translated into pedagogical practice, given limited resources, skills and materials? Do we have a sufficient range of differentiated teaching methods to take advantage of the differences we see in children's abilities? Can we even imagine what it might mean for a teacher to be overseeing the personalised learning of 30 children under their purview?

TECHNOLOGY

One answer to the personalisation challenge is technology, since computerised adaptive content can respond to the individual pro-pensities of each learner, moving them to more challenging mate-rial only when they have mastered what has come before. With developments in artificial intelligence and machine learning, some very sophisticated systems are coming on stream. We also witness the immersive attention some students pay to commercial video games – and over very long periods of time – and wonder if there are lessons here for educational games. Currently, they are lagging behind; less investment in their development means they are a long way behind in quality, and focus more on content rather than the game dynamics which are so important to the success of their commercial cousins. This situation might change. The years of the pandemic focused minds on remote learning, with wins and losses. The period saw woeful increases in social inequality as many lacked access to devices, networks and financial resources. But the hope is that it might in the longer term lead to games developers turning their attention, potentially backed by governments or others, to developing games that not only trigger engagement and curiosity as successfully as existing games, but with the added dimension of educational content.

Other developments in technology are moving forward apace. Projects like the electroencephalograms (EEGs) pilot study in China highlighted in Chapter 1, potentially give students (and their teachers) greater insight into the workings of their brains – with the hope that this allows them to maximise times of most efficient information processing. The fact that data are also shared beyond classrooms – to parents and government agencies – raises many ethical concerns. But neurofeedback techniques which allow individuals to gradually learn to recognise and adapt their thinking approaches as they learn hold promise.

The bigger questions concerning the effects of the use of smart phones will, given their ubiquity, continue to be raised over the coming years and decades and longitudinal data tracking effects over time will be increasingly available. So far, the data suggest that the most concerning effects of these devices are their association with disrupted sleep – greater phone use being associated with reduced quantity and quality of sleep – and with poorer mental health, including anxiety and depression, particularly for adolescents. Yet the facility that social media provided for isolated teenagers to maintain social connections during the pandemic shows that the impact of technology has to be viewed in a balanced way.

Another aspect of technological development is in improvements in research methods. New technology, such as eye tracking, mouse tracking, portable versions of EEG and other headsets which measure brain activity, are all being increasingly used. They have the benefit of allowing brains to be studied in more real-world settings: the home or the classroom, rather than the obviously artificial environment of an MRI scanner.

GETTING EMOTIONAL

Our emotions shape our brains. A better understanding and appreciation of the role of emotions in learning offer great potential for improving outcomes. We know that stress is associated with the emotion of threat and have seen that the relationship between stress and learning is complex. A certain amount of stress can help learning, but excess or chronic stress can be highly detrimental. Positive emotions can also be some of the most powerful learning catalysts. If maximising students' emotional and social experience of learning starts to be considered of primary importance, much else follows: if students can build positive learner identities in a safe and purposeful environment, they will believe their contribution is valuable and it will feel relevant; this in turn is an important trigger for motivation with the potential for a highly productive virtuous circle.

The 'eureka' that is associated with new concepts being grasped is another very powerful promoter of learning; if students get a taste of this at a young age, it shows them that learning can be satisfying and pleasurable.

Emotional regulation is one of the most crucial skills for all students to master, and teachers need to understand how to build and encourage self-regulation as it changes dramatically over development. Learning successfully means being able to cope with setbacks, having the flexibility to change tack, being resilient to failure and being able to maintain attention and focus on demand. These are difficult skills. A focus on helping students to grasp, practise and maintain them is one of the most important jobs teachers can do.

ADOLESCENCE

Until recently, it was thought that most brain development had taken place by the time we reached puberty. Over the past two decades, neuroimaging evidence from brain scans has shown how far that is from the true picture. The big differences in the teenage brain are in attention, motivation and reward. Teenagers are challenged by new environments, involving novel social negotiations, experimental behaviours and thrill seeking, and have new goals – again often social goals of impressing their peers. So there is a burst of new learning, particularly in those areas most plastic at that point, such as prefrontal cortex. There are inconsistencies in behaviour (as parents of teens know) and once changes to goals, rewards and motivation are induced by changing hormones and neurotransmitters, this can reveal underlying weaknesses that put adolescents and young adults at higher risk for certain mental health problems.

So some areas of adolescent brains are particularly plastic, meaning that, with the right environment, adolescence is potentially a very productive time for learning. However, we are still uncovering what exactly constitutes this 'right environment'. We know that during adolescence, the prefrontal cortex (which controls attention and behaviour, sitting at the top of chain for abstract and complex thought and for future planning) is still developing. The emotional system, under the influence of a wash of puberty hormones, is also rapidly changing. These altered dynamics create conditions for positive or negative feedback loops, as teenagers bloom or veer off the rails. The combination lies behind the description of adolescence as a time of 'high horsepower, poor steering' – young people have high cognitive capacity but are still relatively emotionally immature.

It is worth noting that juvenile behaviour, rather than being a uniquely human phenomenon, is found across species. It has likely been selected by evolution and therefore optimised to some extent. If teens do apparently crazy things, they do it for evolutionary reasons not because their brains aren't working properly! For example, taking risks might be to gain a good position in the social dominance hierarchy but this means learning fast, and on the job, about what constitutes a sensible level of risk. Some will get it wrong. The role of parents and caregivers in this time is not to remove all risk taking, since that will delay the dawning of wisdom, but to protect young people from the worst adverse effects of risk, particularly when those involve drugs, alcohol and driving – and to tune in to young people's mental well-being, since suicide is still the highest cause of death in this age group (Office for National Statistics, 2018).

Our evolving knowledge of adolescent brain changes will shape what goes on in classrooms. We now know that the adolescent brain responds differently to rewards than adults. Since instant gratification is a key goal for adolescents, they are much more responsive to rewards in the here and now than promised future rewards. They are more highly sensitive to social and emotional cues – both of which can have positive or negative consequences, depending how they are used. Risk-taking, sensation-seeking and heightened social awareness can all, with careful guidance, be used as positive factors in the classroom, for example, by exploiting opportunities for collaborative learning, peer feedback, rearranging the physical space of classrooms to make them less teacher-centric and by being highly attuned and sensitive to the effects of feedback, positive or negative.

Adolescence is a unique time in that young people have a great ability to shape the development of their own brains. They are old enough to understand themselves and the world and to think about their thinking. Their emotions mean they can be intensely engaged and motivated. They are sufficiently autonomous to make their own choices. Helping adolescents understand what is going on inside their own heads during this phase of seismic remodelling could prove, reflexively, a powerful tool for its development.

BOX 9.2   NEURODEVELOPMENTAL CONDITIONS

Neuroscience has an important contribution to make to understanding the brain basis of what researchers call neurodevelopmental disorders – conditions associated with functional challenges in learning skills, such as those required in education. Box 9.3 refers to language choices in how we speak about these conditions. We talked about the specific cases of dyslexia and dyscalculia in Chapter 8 but there are many other conditions which affect learning, including autism (sometimes also called autism spectrum disorder (ASD)), attention deficit/hyperactivity disorder (ADHD), motor disorders, genetic disorders, and intellectual disability. How can educational neuroscience help here?

Most neurodevelopmental conditions arise through complex, multi-component interactions between genes and the environment.

When it comes to behavioural conditions that impact children's ability to learn, there is no single gene *for* a particular condition. Rather, many small effects from many different genes manifest through different interactions with many different features of the environment to bring about a range of varieties and strengths of a condition. Many of these conditions are 'spectrums', with a broad range of manifestations. This wide individual variation makes it complicated to see what is going on in the brain, but with time, not impossible.

Let's take the example of ADHD. Children with the condition have trouble controlling their attention, and difficulty with organisation and regulation – of emotions, of behaviour, of thoughts. Their flexible attention can also have benefits, for example, in creative thinking. There are many different aspects to attention (as we discussed in Chapter 5). In ADHD, children have trouble with brain networks that sustain attention (leading to difficulty focusing especially over longer periods of time) but the attention networks responsible for *alerting* the brain are often *too* active, meaning they are constantly being called to respond to cues from the environment, which can easily become overwhelming. In the brain, ADHD is thought to be caused by problems with *inhibitory control* which is the brain's 'braking system'. Activating inhibitory control helps to dampen certain thought pathways to concentrate attention on others. Neuroimaging of those with ADHD shows variation in the typical patterns of connectivity between different brain regions, and those with the condition often also have altered levels of dopamine and noradrenaline, two of the brain's most important neurotransmitters, which affect motivation and alertness.

Given that attention skills predict performance for all children, it is no surprise that those with attention problems as in ADHD tend to have poorer academic outcomes. ADHD can be treated pharmacologically, for example, with psychostimulants that boost dopamine, or with behavioural interventions. These interventions might be simple things, such as reducing the level of distraction in the classroom, for example, seating children to minimise visual distractions; ensuring instructions are clear, repeated and kept visible; breaking long tasks into small chunks; explicit scheduling; setting goals and giving rewards in short, manageable amounts. Interventions to train self-control and develop problem-solving skills to help children regulate their thoughts and actions can also be helpful.

Many myths exist about neurodevelopmental conditions. We would encourage anyone interested to look at the Centre for Educational Neuroscience resource *NeuroSENse* for accurate information (see Resources).

SPECIAL EDUCATIONAL NEEDS AND DISABILITIES

Educational neuroscience has an important role to play in developing an evidence-based pedagogical approach for students with special educational needs and disabilities (SEND). It has already made a significant contribution to improving understanding of the causes of dyslexia and offering potential for intervention at a very young age. Even at birth, electrical activity in the brain can be used to predict whether a child is at risk of dyslexia, based on responsivity to auditory signals. Neuroprognosis in the early years can go further and help suggest which types of intervention are likely to be most beneficial to which children, depending on their underlying patterns of brain connectivity. Similarly, neuroscience has contributed important evidence to help understand the brain basis of dyscalculia, deafness, attention deficit disorder (ADD) and autism, as well as genetic disorders, such as Williams Syndrome and Down syndrome. There is, as well, a growing awareness among researchers of the importance of recognizing neurodiversity and placing the practical needs of children with these conditions at the heart of research efforts (see Box 9.2 Neurodevelopmental conditions).

BOX 9.3   NEURODEVELOPMENTAL DIVERSITY

There is a very high prevalence of neurodevelopmental diversity; 16–30 per cent of children have trouble learning, whether or not they have a clinically diagnosed disorder. Diagnosis itself can be very problematic: there is high overlap of symptoms in different conditions, as well as high levels of comorbidity (that is, children with more than one diagnosis) while, at the same time, many children with some or all those same symptoms never receive any diagnosis.

Historically, named conditions have been at the heart of thinking about developmental difficulties, with research focused on finding the 'core deficit' which underlies them. In reality, the array of profiles of deficits suggests there is sometimes as much dividing those with the same condition as uniting them and few conditions have produced coherent theoretical models to explain the mechanisms which cause them. Because it is hard to find 'pure', well-defined groups to investigate these putative core deficits, many studies end up having small samples. They exclude many children on the basis that they are not of the 'correct' sample (e.g., ruling out those with multiple diagnoses), failing to account for the reality that most conditions are characterised by broad symptom spectrums. Measurement tools often lack a theoretical basis to describe the full group and many neuroimaging studies are based on adults rather than children, which ignores developmental aspects.

There are many ways in which this model of research is not ideal. Some suggest a new *transdiagnostic* approach is desirable and achievable, given new technological advances for the complex analyses involved. The focus would be on shared symptoms rather than common diagnoses. Studies would include children with different or multiple diagnoses who share similar symptom profiles; more data sharing would mean increased sample sizes and new data analysis tools – statistical tools, network analysis and computer models – can better capture complex relationships, that is, to represent the variety of actual struggling learners. The key implication for interventions is to target the *need*, rather than the diagnostic group.

It is too early to say whether affected children and families would be better served by this change of approach, but it has a strong theoretical basis. The change might also signal a shift in focus away from the language of 'deficits' and 'disorders'. There is no firm scientific reason to concentrate only on negative aspects of conditions and there are plenty of reasons for *not* doing so. The more positive aspects of conditions often offer the base material for intervention on the problematic symptoms, such as when images are used to supplement words in dyslexia, or technologies, such as virtual reality environments, are used to help those with autism. This shift in language and emphasis is likely to have benefits in reducing social stigma and perhaps even reducing the considerable mental health burden carried by those with 'disorder' labels.

BRAIN-BASED OR EVIDENCE-BASED?

Educational neuroscience walks in step with the broader objective of shifting education to a more evidence-based approach. What characterises the educational neuroscience endeavour is the need to understand *how things work* – to really get to grips with the mechanisms of learning, in all its complexity. As we have said, this means that much of the early work likely involves refinements of current practices rather than wholesale changes to them. We gave the example of spaced learning, long been known to be beneficial, as a practice for which understanding *how* it works facilitates being more specific about the details – what degree of spacing, repeated how often, for which types of learning, with retrieval how? We drew a parallel with medicine: people have known for 400 years that chewing the bark of a cinchona tree helps treat malaria. People of the time knew 'It works.' But now that we understand much more about the active ingredient in cinchona (quinine), we can specify the dose, improve the means of administration, specify the schedule, understand, and treat side effects, calculate the costs and benefits of prevention vs treatment, find alternative drugs that work in the same way as quinine such as chloroquine, derive treatment options for malaria that shows quinine or chloroquine resistance, and so on.

The point is that just because something works doesn't mean it can't be improved by understanding how it works. That is educational neuroscience in a nutshell.

RESOURCES

We hope this book has given you a taste of what educational neuroscience is all about. If you would like to continue your journey, we hope the following recommendations will help to guide you. The first is a recent publication edited by researchers at the Centre for Educational Neuroscience. It takes a similar starting point to this book but goes into more depth. Following this are recommendations for books which go into more detail about specific areas we have covered in this book, including the emotions, learning, reading, mindset, maths, the social brain, adolescence, and more. Then there are recommendations for online resources – websites, blogs, videos – for teachers and researchers interested in the brain. We wish you a pleasant journey!

Thomas, M. S. C., Mareschal, D., & **Dumontheil, I.** **(2020)**. *Educational neuroscience: Development across the life span*. **Routledge**.

This book brings together the latest knowledge on the development of educational neuroscience from a life-span perspective, offering state-of-the-art, authoritative research findings and providing evidence-based recommendations for classroom practice.

Four main themes are explored. The first is individual differences, or what makes children perform better or worse in the classroom. The second is the nature of individual differences at different stages in development, from early years into adulthood. The third addresses cognitive enhancement, summarising research that has investigated activities that might give general benefits to cognition. And the fourth considers the translation of research findings into classroom practices, discussing broader ethical issues raised by educational neuroscience,

DOI: 10.4324/9781003185642-10

and what teachers need to know about neuroscience to enhance their day-to-day practice. The book is essential reading for researchers and graduate students of educational psychology, developmental science, developmental psychology, and cognitive psychology, especially those specialising in emotion regulation.

BOOKS

Amthor, F. (2016). Neuroscience for dummies. John Wiley & Sons.

Barrett, L. F. (2018). How emotions are made: The secret life of the brain. Pan.

Blakemore, S. (2018). Inventing ourselves: The secret life of the teenage brain. Transworld Publishers Ltd.

Blakemore, S., & Frith, U. (2005). The learning brain: Lessons for education. Blackwell Publishing, especially pp. vi, 216.

Carter, R. (2019). The brain book: An illustrated guide to its structure, functions, and disorders. Dorling Kindersley Ltd.

Churches, R., & Dommett, E. (2016). Teacher-led research: Designing and implementing randomised controlled trials and other forms of experimental research. Crown House Publishing.

Churches, R., Dommett, E., & Devonshire, I. (2017). Neuroscience for teachers: Applying research evidence from brain science. Crown House Publishing Ltd.

Coleman, J. (2021). The teacher and the teenage brain. Routledge.

Dehaene, S. (2010). Reading in the brain: The new science of how we read. Penguin USA.

Dehaene, S. (2011). The number sense: How the mind creates mathematics (Rev. ed.). Oxford University Press, USA.Dehaene, S. (2021). How we learn: Why brains learn better than any machine… for now. Penguin.

Dweck, C. (2006). Mindset: The new psychology of success. Random House Digital, Inc.

Fischer, K. W., & Immordino-Yang, M. H. (2007). The Jossey-Bass reader on the brain and learning. Jossey-Bass.

Geake, J. (2009). The brain at school: Educational neuroscience in the classroom. McGraw-Hill Education (UK).

Hattie, J. (2008). Visible learning: A synthesis of over 800 meta-analyses relating to achievement. Routledge.

Heyes, C. (2018). Cognitive gadgets: The cultural evolution of thinking. Harvard University Press.

Kahneman, D. (2012). Thinking, fast and slow. Penguin.

OECD. (2007). Understanding the brain: The birth of a learning science. OECD.

Schwartz, D. L., Tsang, J. M., & Blair, K. R. (2016). The ABCs of how we learn. Norton.

Sousa, D. A. (2010). Mind, brain, & education: Neuroscience implications for the classroom. Solution Tree Press.

Sousa, D. A. (2011). How the brain learns (4th ed.). Corwin.

Thomas, M. S. C., Mareschal, D., & Dumontheil, I. (2020). Educational neuroscience: Development across the life span. Routledge.

Tokuhama-Espinosa, T. (2010). Mind, brain, and education science: A comprehensive guide to the new brain-based teaching. W. W. Norton & Company.

Tokuhama-Espinosa, T. (2014). Making classrooms better: 50 practical applications of mind, brain, and education science. W. W. Norton & Company.

WEBSITES/BLOGS

Resources, events and information about educational neuroscience: http://www.educationalneuroscience.org.uk/.

Accessible introduction to the brain's workings, produced by the Centre for Educational Neuroscience: http://howthebrainworks.science.

A collection of articles about the brain written by neuroscientists for students and teachers: https://kids.frontiersin.org/collections/10207/everything-you-and-your-teachers-need-to-know-about-the-learning-brain.

Practical advice for teachers based on cognitive science evidence: https://www.learningscientists.org/.

Education Endowment Foundation's toolkit of evidence for effective, scientifically evaluated school interventions in the UK: https://educationendowmentfoundation.org.uk/education-evidence/teaching-learning-toolkit.

A similar set of resources for the US from the 'What Works Clearing House': https://ies.ed.gov/ncee/wwc/.

Learnus is a Think Tank that supports the engagement and dialogue between educators and researchers working in the field of educational neuroscience: https://www.learnus.co.uk/.

UK research resources from schools which are part of the Research Schools Network: https://researchschool.org.uk/. We would also recommend Huntington research school's resources as part of this network https://researchschool.org.uk/huntington/news.

Neuroscience blog centred on the emotional brain: https://lisafeldmanbarrett.com/articles/.

The Harvard Centre on the Developing Child, scientific research supporting child development: https://developingchild.harvard.edu/.

2-minute guides, pictures, and videos to all the parts of the brain: https://neuroscientificallychallenged.com/.

International Mind, Brain and Education Society website: www.imbes.org.

Two excellent blogs from people who have been both teachers and educational neuroscience researchers: https://hobbolog.wordpress.com/ and https://overpractised.wordpress.com/.

Expert resources on development, learning and education: https://bold.expert/.

Great visual guides to teaching strategies produced by a former headteacher and excellent graphic artist: https://www.olicav.com.

Lisa Feldman Barrett's cinematic lecture on 'How emotions are made': https://www.youtube.com/watch?v=0rbyC5m557I.

The Psychologist, the magazine of the British Psychological Society, has many interesting articles about educational neuroscience, such as this one: https://thepsychologist.bps.org.uk/volume-29/october-2016/learning-educational-neuroscience.

Neuroscience for kids: resources for students and teachers: http://faculty.washington.edu/chudler/neurok.html.

Video of a talk by Paul Howard-Jones on neuroscience and education, asking 'How can we play, learn and be more creative?': https://www.youtube.com/watch?v=docSZBq3juY.

Short video introduction to educational neuroscience by Professor Michael Thomas: https://www.youtube.com/watch?v=2uK3d9hL-IQ.

REFERENCES

Aguilar, L., Walton, G., & Wieman, C. (2014). Psychological insights for improved physics. *Physics Today*, 67 (5), 43–49. https://doi.org/10.1063/PT.3.2383.

Altimus, C. M., Marlin, B. J., Charalambakis, N. E., Colón-Rodríguez, A., Glover, E. J., Izbicki, P., Johnson, A., Lourenco, M. V., Makinson, R. A., McQuail, J., Obeso, I., Padilla-Coreano, N., & Wells, M. F. (2020). The next 50 years of neuroscience. *Journal of Neuroscience*, 40 (1), 101–106. https://doi.org/10.1523/JNEUROSCI.0744-19.2019.

Amso, D., & Scerif, G. (2015). The attentive brain: Insights from developmental cognitive neuroscience. *Nature Reviews Neuroscience*, 16 (10), 606–619. https://doi.org/10.1038/nrn4025.

Amthor, F. (2016). *Neuroscience for dummies*. John Wiley & Sons.

Arnsten, A. F. T. (2009). Stress signalling pathways that impair prefrontal cortex structure and function. *Nature Reviews Neuroscience*, 10 (6), 410–422. https://doi.org/10.1038/nrn2648.

Asbury, K., & Plomin, R. (2013). *G is for genes: The impact of genetics on education and achievement*. John Wiley & Sons.

Asfestani, M. A., Brechtmann, V., Santiago, J., Peter, A., Born, J., & Feld, G. B. (2020). Consolidation of reward memory during sleep does not require dopaminergic activation. *Journal of Cognitive Neuroscience*, 32 (9), 1688–1703. https://doi.org/10.1162/jocn_a_01585.

Astle, D. E., & Fletcher-Watson, S. (2020). Beyond the core-deficit hypothesis in developmental disorders. *Current Directions in Psychological Science*, 29 (5), 431–437. https://doi.org/10.1177/0963721420925518.

Astle, D. E., Holmes, J., Kievit, R., & Gathercole, S. E. (2021). Annual research review: The transdiagnostic revolution in neurodevelopmental disorders. *Journal of Child Psychology and Psychiatry*. https://doi.org/10.1111/jcpp.13481.

Baddeley, A. (2003). Working memory: Looking back and looking forward. *Nature Reviews Neuroscience*, 4 (10), 829–839. https://doi.org/10.1038/nrn1201.

Baldwin, D. A., Markman, E. M., Bill, B., Desjardins, R. N., Irwin, J. M., & Tidball, G. (1996). Infants' reliance on a social criterion for establishing word-object relations. *Child Development*, 67 (6), 3135–3153. https://doi.org/10.1111/j.1467-8624.1996.tb01906.x.

Banich, M. T., & Compton, R. J. (2018). *Cognitive neuroscience*. Cambridge University Press.

Barrett, L. F. (2018). *How emotions are made: The secret life of the brain*. Pan.

Barrett, L. F. (2021). Why chimpanzees don't hold elections: The power of social reality. *Undark Magazine*. https://undark.org/2021/01/01/book-excerpt-seven-and-a-half-lessons-about-the-brain/.

Barsalou, L. W. (2008). Grounded cognition. *Annual Review of Psychology*, 59 (1), 617–645. https://doi.org/10.1146/annurev.psych.59.103006.093639.

Beckingham, K. (2020). What's next for personalised learning in education? Education Technology. https://edtechnology.co.uk/latest-news/rise-personalised-learning-education/.

Bell, D., & Darlington, H. M. (2020). Educational neuroscience: So what does it mean in the classroom? In M. S. C. Thomas, D. Mareschal, & I. Dumontheil (Eds.), *Educational neuroscience*. Routledge.

Bell, D., Mareschal, D., & Unlocke Team (2021). UnLocke-ing learning in maths and science: The role of cognitive inhibition in developing counter-intuitive concepts. *Journal of Emergent Science*, 20, 19–31.

Benasich, A. A., Choudhury, N. A., Realpe-Bonilla, T., & Roesler, C. P. (2014). Plasticity in developing brain: Active auditory exposure impacts prelinguistic acoustic mapping. *Journal of Neuroscience*, 34 (40), 13349–13363. https://doi.org/10.1523/JNEUROSCI.0972-14.2014.

Benjamin, A. S., & Tullis, J. (2010). What makes distributed practice effective? *Cognitive Psychology*, 61 (3), 228–247. https://doi.org/10.1016/j.cogpsych.2010.05.004.

Bialystok, E., Craik, F. I. M., & Freedman, M. (2007). Bilingualism as a protection against the onset of symptoms of dementia. *Neuropsychologia*, 45 (2), 459–464. https://doi.org/10.1016/j.Neuropsychologia.2006.10.009.

Blackburn, K., & Schirillo, J. (2012). Emotive hemispheric differences measured in real-life portraits using pupil diameter and subjective aesthetic preferences. *Experimental Brain Research*, 219 (4), 447–455. https://doi.org/10.1007/s00221-012-3091-y.

Blackwell, L. S., Trzesniewski, K. H., & Dweck, C. S. (2007). Implicit theories of intelligence predict achievement across an adolescent transition: A longitudinal study and an intervention. *Child Development*, 78 (1), 246–263.

Blakemore, S.-J. (2018a). Avoiding social risk in adolescence. *Current Directions in Psychological Science*, 27 (2), 116–122. https://doi.org/10.1177/0963721417738144.

Blakemore, S.-J. (2018b). *Inventing ourselves: The secret life of the teenage brain.* Transworld Publishers Ltd.

Blakemore, S.-J., & Frith, U. (2005). *The learning brain: Lessons for education* (pp. vi,216). Blackwell Publishing.

Blakemore, S.-J., Winston, J., & Frith, U. (2004). Social cognitive neuroscience: Where are we heading? *Trends in Cognitive Sciences,* 8 (5), 216–222. https://doi.org/10.1016/j.tics.2004.03.012.

Bloom, P. (2002). *How children learn the meanings of words.* MIT Press.

Bostrom, N. (2015). *Superintelligence: Paths, dangers, strategies* (unabridged ed.). Audible Studios on Brilliance Audio.

Boysen, S. T., & Capaldi, E. J. (2014). *The development of numerical competence: Animal and human models.* Psychology Press.

Brockington, G., Balardin, J. B., Zimeo Morais, G. A., Malheiros, A., Lent, R., Moura, L. M., & Sato, J. R. (2018). From the laboratory to the classroom: The potential of functional near-infrared spectroscopy in educational neuroscience. *Frontiers in Psychology,* 9, 1840. https://doi.org/10.3389/fpsyg.2018.01840.

Brookman-Byrne, A., Mareschal, D., Tolmie, A. K., & Dumontheil, I. (2018). Inhibitory control and counterintuitive science and maths reasoning in adolescence. *PLoS ONE,* 13 (6), e0198973. https://doi.org/10.1371/journal.pone.0198973.

Brown, S., Cockett, P., & Yuan, Y. (2019). The neuroscience of *Romeo and Juliet*: An fMRI study of acting. *Royal Society Open Science,* 6 (3), 181908. https://doi.org/10.1098/rsos.181908.

Bruer, J. T. (1997). Education and the brain: A bridge too far. *Educational Researcher,* 26 (8), 4–16. https://doi.org/10.3102/0013189X026008004.

Butterworth, B. (2005). The development of arithmetical abilities. *Journal of Child Psychology and Psychiatry,* 46 (1), 3–18. https://doi.org/10.1111/j.1469-7610.2004.00374.x.

Butterworth, B., Varma, S., & Laurillard, D. (2011). Dyscalculia: From brain to education. *Science,* 332 (6033), 1049–1053. https://doi.org/10.1126/science.1201536.

Carter, R. (2019). *The brain book: An illustrated guide to its structure, functions, and disorders.* Dorling Kindersley Ltd.

Cepeda, N. J., Pashler, H., Vul, E., Wixted, J. T., & Rohrer, D. (2006). Distributed practice in verbal recall tasks: A review and quantitative synthesis. *Psychological Bulletin,* 132 (3), 354–380. https://doi.org/10.1037/0033-2909.132.3.354.

Churches, R., & Dommett, E. (2016). *Teacher-led research: Designing and implementing randomised controlled trials and other forms of experimental research.* Crown House Publishing.

Churches, R., Dommett, E., & Devonshire, I. (2017). *Neuroscience for teachers: Applying research evidence from brain science.* Crown House Publishing Ltd.

Clark, L. (2012, November 12). Chess returns to the timetable: Schools reintroduce game in attempt to improve children's brainpower. *Mail Online*. Available at: https://www.dailymail.co.uk/news/article-2232014/Chess-returns-schools-boost-childrens-brainpower.html.

Cohen Kadosh, K., & Johnson, M. H. (2007). Developing a cortex specialized for face perception. *Trends in Cognitive Sciences*, 11 (9), 367–369. https://doi.org/10.1016/j.tics.2007.06.007.

Coleman, J. (2021). *The teacher and the teenage brain*. Routledge.

Cottingham, S. (n.d.). Evidence for educators. Blog. https://overpractised.wordpress.com/category/neuroscience/.

Csibra, G. (2003). Teleological and referential understanding of action in infancy. *Philosophical Transactions of the Royal Society of London B: Biological Sciences*, 358 (1431), 447–458. https://doi.org/10.1098/rstb.2002.1235.

Dahlstrom, M. F. (2014). Using narratives and storytelling to communicate science with nonexpert audiences. *Proceedings of the National Academy of Sciences*, 111 (Suppl. 4), 13614–13620. https://doi.org/10.1073/pnas.1320645111.

Daily Mail. (2009). How learning to play a musical instrument can boost your IQ. *Mail Online*. Available at: https://www.dailymail.co.uk/sciencetech/article-1223431/How-learning-play-musical-instrument-boost-IQ.html.

Damasio, A. R. (2006). *Descartes' error*. Random House.

Davidson, M. C., Amso, D., Anderson, L. C., & Diamond, A. (2006). Development of cognitive control and executive functions from 4 to 13 years: Evidence from manipulations of memory, inhibition, and task switching. *Neuropsychologia*, 44 (11), 2037–2078. https://doi.org/10.1016/j.Neuropsychologia.2006.02.006.

Dehaene, S. (2010). *Reading in the brain: The new science of how we read* (illustrated ed.). Penguin USA.

Dehaene, S. (2011). *The number sense: How the mind creates mathematics*. (rev. ed.). Oxford University Press.

Dehaene, S. (2021). *How we learn: The new science of education and the brain*. Penguin.

Dehaene, S., & Cohen, L. (2007). Cultural recycling of cortical maps. *Neuron*, 56 (2), 384–398. https://doi.org/10.1016/j.neuron.2007.10.004.

Dehaene, S., Cohen, L., Sigman, M., & Vinckier, F. (2005). The neural code for written words: A proposal. *Trends in Cognitive Sciences*, 9 (7), 335–341. https://doi.org/10.1016/j.tics.2005.05.004.

Dehaene, S., & Dehaene-Lambertz, G. (2016). Is the brain prewired for letters? *Nature Neuroscience*, 19 (9), 1192–1193. https://doi.org/10.1038/nn.4369.

De Klerk, C. C. J. M., Johnson, M. H., & Southgate, V. (2015). An EEG study on the somatotopic organisation of sensorimotor cortex activation during action execution and observation in infancy. *Developmental Cognitive Neuroscience*, 15, 1–10. Scopus. https://doi.org/10.1016/j.dcn.2015.08.004.

Diekelmann, S., & Born, J. (2010). The memory function of sleep. *Nature Reviews Neuroscience*, 11 (2), 114–126. https://doi.org/10.1038/nrn2762.

Dockrell, J. E., Braisby, N., & Best, R. M. (2007). Children's acquisition of science terms: Simple exposure is insufficient. *Learning and Instruction*, 17 (6), 577–594. https://doi.org/10.1016/j.learninstruc.2007.09.005.

Donaldson, M. I. (2017). Teaching and learning from mistakes: Teachers' responses to student mistakes in the kindergarten classroom. https://dash.harvard.edu/handle/1/33052857.

Duckworth, A. (2016). *Grit: The power of passion and perseverance.* Scribner.

Duckworth, A. (2017). *Grit: Why passion and resilience are the secrets to success* (1st ed.). Vermilion.

Dweck, C. (2006). *Mindset: The new psychology of success.* Random House Digital, Inc.

Education Endowment Foundation. (2018). Guidance report: Metacognition and self-regulated learning. Available at: educationendowmentfoundation.org.uk/education.

Education Endowment Foundation. (n.d.). Guidance reports. Available at: https://educationendowmentfoundation.org.uk/education-evidence/guidance-reports. (accessed 21 September 2021).

Elfenbein, H. A., & Ambady, N. (2002). On the universality and cultural specificity of emotion recognition: A meta-analysis. *Psychological Bulletin*, 128 (2), 203–235. https://doi.org/10.1037/0033-2909.128.2.203.

Erickson, K. I., Voss, M. W., Prakash, R. S., Basak, C., Szabo, A., Chaddock, L., Kim, J. S., Heo, S., Alves, H., White, S. M., Wojcicki, T. R., Mailey, E., Vieira, V. J., Martin, S. A., Pence, B. D., Woods, J. A., McAuley, E., & Kramer, A. F. (2011). Exercise training increases size of hippocampus and improves memory. *Proceedings of the National Academy of Sciences*, 108 (7), 3017–3022. https://doi.org/10.1073/pnas.1015950108.

Evans, G. W., & Kim, P. (2013). Childhood poverty, chronic stress, self-regulation, and coping. *Child Development Perspectives*, 7 (1), 43–48. https://doi.org/10.1111/cdep.12013.

Faber, N. S., Douglas, T., Heise, F., & Hewstone, M. (2015). Cognitive enhancement and motivation enhancement: An empirical comparison of intuitive judgments. *AJOB Neuroscience*, 6 (1), 18–20. https://doi.org/10.1080/21507740.2014.991847.

Feiler, J. B., & Stabio, M. E. (2018). Three pillars of educational neuroscience from three decades of literature. *Trends in Neuroscience and Education*, 13, 17–25. https://doi.org/10.1016/j.tine.2018.11.001.

Fields, D. R. (2005). Making memories stick. *Scientific American*, 292 (2), 74–81.

Fischer, K. W., Goswami, U., Geake, J., & the Task Force on the Future of Educational Neuroscience. (2010). The future of educational neuroscience.

Mind, Brain, and Education, 4 (2), 68–80. https://doi.org/10.1111/j.1751-228X. 2010.01086.x.

Fischer, K. W., & Immordino-Yang, M. H. (2007). *The Jossey-Bass reader on the brain and learning.* Jossey-Bass.

Forbes, S. C., Holroyd-Leduc, J. M., Poulin, M. J., & Hogan, D. B. (2015). Effect of nutrients, dietary supplements and vitamins on cognition: A systematic review and meta-analysis of randomized controlled trials. *Canadian Geriatrics Journal*, 18 (4), 231–245. https://doi.org/10.5770/cgj.18.189.

Forrester, G. S., Davis, R., Mareschal, D., Malatesta, G., & Todd, B. K. (2019). The left cradling bias: An evolutionary facilitator of social cognition? *Cortex*, 118, 116–131. https://doi.org/10.1016/j.cortex.2018.05.011.

Foulkes, L., & Blakemore, S.-J. (2016). Is there heightened sensitivity to social reward in adolescence? *Current Opinion in Neurobiology*, 40, 81–85. https:// doi.org/10.1016/j.conb.2016.06.016.

Frank, C., Land, W. M., Popp, C., & Schack, T. (2014). Mental representation and mental practice: Experimental investigation on the functional links between motor memory and motor imagery. *PLoS ONE*, 9 (4), e95175. https://doi.org/10.1371/journal.pone.0095175.

Frith, U., & Frith, C. (2010). The social brain: Allowing humans to boldly go where no other species has been. *Philosophical Transactions of the Royal Society B: Biological Sciences*, 365 (1537), 165–176. https://doi.org/10.1098/rstb.2009. 0160.

Gabi, M., Neves, K., Masseron, C., Ribeiro, P. F. M., Ventura-Antunes, L., Torres, L., Mota, B., Kaas, J. H., & Herculano-Houzel, S. (2016). No relative expansion of the number of prefrontal neurons in primate and human evolution. *Proceedings of the National Academy of Sciences of the United States of America*, 113 (34), 9617–9622. https://doi.org/10.1073/pnas.1610178113.

Gabrieli, J. D. E. (2009). Dyslexia: A new synergy between education and cognitive neuroscience. *Science*, 325 (5938), 280–283. https://doi.org/10. 1126/science.1171999.

Galetzka, C. (2017). The story so far: How embodied cognition advances our understanding of meaning-making. *Frontiers in Psychology*, 8. https://www. frontiersin.org/article/10.3389/fpsyg.2017.01315.

Gardner, M., & Steinberg, L. (2005). Peer influence on risk taking, risk preference, and risky decision making in adolescence and adulthood: An experimental study. *Developmental Psychology*, 41 (4), 625–635. https://doi. org/10.1037/0012-1649.41.4.625.

Geake, J. (2009). *The brain at school: Educational neuroscience in the classroom.* McGraw-Hill Education (UK).

Gilbert, C. D., Sigman, M., & Crist, R. E. (2001). The neural basis of perceptual learning. *Neuron*, 31 (5), 681–697. https://doi.org/10.1016/ s0896-6273(01)00424-x.

Gilboa, A., & Verfaellie, M. (2010). Introduction—telling it like it isn't: The cognitive neuroscience of confabulation. *Journal of the International Neuropsychological Society*, 16 (6), 961–966.

Goldacre, B. (2013). Building evidence into education. Available at: http://thesendhub.co.uk/wp-content/uploads/2016/09/building-evidence-into-education.pdf.

Goswami, U. (2008). The development of reading across languages. *Annals of the New York Academy of Sciences*, 1145 (1), 1–12. https://doi.org/10.1196/annals.1416.018.

Goswami, U. (2009). Mind, brain, and literacy: Biomarkers as usable knowledge for education. *Mind, Brain, and Education*, 3 (3), 176–184. https://doi.org/10.1111/j.1751-228X.2009.01068.x.

Gotlieb, R. J. M., Pollack, C., Younger, J. W., Toomarian, E. Y., Allaire-Duquette, G., & Mariager, N. M. (2019). Next steps for mind, brain, and education: Strengthening early-career development. *Mind, Brain, and Education*, 13 (3), 120–132. https://doi.org/10.1111/mbe.12197.

Gould, S. J., & Vrba, E. S. (1982). Exaptation: A missing term in the science of form. *Paleobiology*, 8 (1), 4–15. https://doi.org/10.1017/S0094837300004310.

Gracia-Bafalluy, M., & Noël, M.-P. (2008). Does finger training increase young children's numerical performance? *Cortex*, 44 (4), 368–375.

Graesser, A. C., & Ottati, V. (1995). *Why stories? Some evidence, questions, and challenges* (p. 132). Lawrence Erlbaum Associates, Inc.

Grantham-McGregor, S. (2005). Can the provision of breakfast benefit school performance? *Food and Nutrition Bulletin*, 26 (Suppl. 2), S144–S158. https://doi.org/10.1177/15648265050262S204.

Greve, A., Cooper, E., Tibon, R., & Henson, R. N. (2019). Knowledge is power: Prior knowledge aids memory for both congruent and incongruent events, but in different ways. *Journal of Experimental Psychology: General*, 148 (2), 325–341. https://doi.org/10.1037/xge0000498.

Grynszpan, O., Weiss, P. L. T., Perez-Diaz, F., & Gal, E. (2014). Innovative technology-based interventions for autism spectrum disorders: A meta-analysis. *Autism*, 18 (4), 346–361. https://doi.org/10.1177/1362361313476767.

Guttorm, T. K., Leppänen, P. H. T., Hämäläinen, J. A., Eklund, K. M., & Lyytinen, H. J. (2010). Newborn event-related potentials predict poorer pre-reading skills in children at risk for dyslexia. *Journal of Learning Disabilities*, 43 (5), 391–401. https://doi.org/10.1177/0022219409345005.

Hackman, D. A., Farah, M. J., & Meaney, M. J. (2010). Socioeconomic status and the brain: Mechanistic insights from human and animal research. *Nature Reviews Neuroscience*, 11 (9), 651–659. https://doi.org/10.1038/nrn2897.

Hanushek, E. A. (2011). Valuing teachers: How much is a good teacher worth? *Education Next*, 11 (3), 40–45.

Hart, L. A. (1999). *Human brain and human learning*. Longman Publishing Group.

Hattie, J. (2003). Teachers make a difference: What is the research evidence? Paper presented at the Australian Conference of Educational Research. http://research.acer.edu.au/research_conference_2005/7.

Hattie, J. (2008). *Visible learning: A synthesis of over 800 meta-analyses relating to achievement*. Routledge. https://doi.org/10.4324/9780203887332.

Heider, F., & Simmel, M. (1944). An experimental study of apparent behavior. *American Journal of Psychology*, 57 (2), 243–259.

Heyes, C. (2018). *Cognitive gadgets: The cultural evolution of thinking*. Harvard University Press. https://doi.org/10.4159/9780674985155.

Hidi, S. (2016). Revisiting the role of rewards in motivation and learning: Implications of neuroscientific research. *Educational Psychology Review*, 28 (1), 61–93. https://doi.org/10.1007/s10648-015-9307-5.

Hirsh, J. B., & Inzlicht, M. (2010). Error-related negativity predicts academic performance. *Psychophysiology*, 47 (1), 192–196. https://doi.org/10.1111/j.1469-8986.2009.00877.x.

Hobbiss, M. H., Massonnié, J., Tokuhama-Espinosa, T., Gittner, A., Sousa Lemos, M. A., Tovazzi, A., Hindley, C., Baker, S., Sumeracki, M. A., Wassenaar, T., & Gous, I. (2019). "UNIFIED": Bridging the researcher-practitioner divide in mind, brain, and education. *Mind, Brain, and Education*, 13 (4), 298–312. https://doi.org/10.1111/mbe.12223.

Hobbiss, M., Sims, S., & Allen, R. (2021). Habit formation limits growth in teacher effectiveness: A review of converging evidence from neuroscience and social science. *Review of Education*, 9 (1), 3–23. https://doi.org/10.1002/rev3.3226.

Hobbolog. (2016a). This confused 'neuro-educationalist' claptrap won't help educational neuroscience. The Hobbolog. Blog. https://hobbolog.wordpress.com/2016/10/12/this-confused-neuro-educationalist-claptrap-wont-help-educational-neuroscience/.

Hobbolog. (2016b). The 'transfer' problem is not a surprise: It's central to how the brain operates. The Hobbolog. Blog. https://hobbolog.wordpress.com/2016/10/25/the-transfer-problem-is-not-a-surprise-its-central-to-how-the-brain-operates/.

Hobbolog. (2017). Pay attention! Why I think it is important to study attention in school children. The Hobbolog. Blog. https://hobbolog.wordpress.com/2017/10/07/pay-attention-why-i-think-it-is-important-to-study-attention-in-school-children/.

Hobbolog. (2020). Attention in the classroom. My 'best bets' from the research. The Hobbolog. Blog. https://hobbolog.wordpress.com/2020/01/30/attention-in-the-classroom-my-best-bets-from-the-research/.

Holmes, J., Guy, J., Kievit, R. A., Bryant, A., Mareva, S., Team, C., & Gathercole, S. E. (2020). Cognitive dimensions of learning in children with problems in attention, learning, and memory. *Journal of Educational Psychology*, 113 (7), 1454. https://doi.org/10.1037/edu0000644.

Horvath, J. C., Donoghue, G. M., Horton, A. J., Lodge, J. M., & Hattie, J. A. C. (2018). On the irrelevance of neuromyths to teacher effectiveness: Comparing neuro-literacy levels amongst award-winning and non-award-winning teachers. *Frontiers in Psychology*, 9, 1666. https://doi.org/10.3389/fpsyg.2018.01666.

Houdé, O., & Borst, G. (2015). Evidence for an inhibitory-control theory of the reasoning brain. *Frontiers in Human Neuroscience*, 9. https://www.frontiersin.org/article/10.3389/fnhum.2015.00148.

Houdé, O., Zago, L., Mellet, E., Moutier, S., Pineau, A., Mazoyer, B., & Tzourio-Mazoyer, N. (2000). Shifting from the perceptual brain to the logical brain: The neural impact of cognitive inhibition training. *Journal of Cognitive Neuroscience*, 12 (5), 721–728. https://doi.org/10.1162/089892900562525.

Howard-Jones, P. A. (2014). Neuroscience and education: Myths and messages. *Nature Reviews Neuroscience*, 15 (12), 817–824. https://doi.org/10.1038/nrn3817.

Howard-Jones, P. A. (2015). Engaging the brain's reward system: The 'Scinapse' Project. *ThInk*. https://thinkneuroscience.wordpress.com/2015/05/15/engaging-the-brains-reward-system-the-sci-napse-project/.

Howard-Jones, P. A., Ioannou, K., Bailey, R., Prior, J., Jay, T., & Yau, S. (2020). Towards a science of teaching and learning for teacher education. In M. S. C. Thomas, D. Mareschal, & I. Dumontheil (Eds.), *Educational neuroscience*. Routledge.

Howard-Jones, P. A., Taylor, J., & Sutton, L. (2002). The effect of play on the creativity of young children during subsequent activity. *Early Child Development and Care*, 172 (4), 323–328. https://doi.org/10.1080/03004430212722.

Howard-Jones, P. A., Varma, S., Ansari, D., Butterworth, B., De Smedt, B., Goswami, U., Laurillard, D., & Thomas, M. S. C. (2016). The principles and practices of educational neuroscience: Comment on Bowers (2016). *Psychological Review*, 123 (5), 620–627. https://doi.org/10.1037/rev0000036.

Howe, C., Tolmie, A., Duchak-Tanner, V., & Rattray, C. (2000). Hypothesis testing in science: Group consensus and the acquisition of conceptual and procedural knowledge. *Learning and Instruction*, 10 (4), 361–391. https://doi.org/10.1016/S0959-4752(00)00004-9.

Hume, D. (1739). *A treatise of human nature*, 3 vols. Reprinted from the original edition (pp. xxiii,709). The Clarendon Press. https://doi.org/10.1037/12868-000.

Illingworth, G., Sharman, R., Harvey, C.-J., Foster, R. G., & Espie, C. A. (2020). The Teensleep study: The effectiveness of a school-based sleep education programme at improving early adolescent sleep. *Sleep Medicine*, X (2), 100011. https://doi.org/10.1016/j.sleepx.2019.100011.

Immordino-Yang, M. H., & Damasio, A. (2007). We feel, therefore we learn: The relevance of affective and social neuroscience to education. *Mind, Brain, and Education*, 1 (1), 3–10. https://doi.org/10.1111/j.1751-228X. 2007.00004.x.

Immordino-Yang, M. H., & Gotlieb, R. J. M. (2020). Understanding emotional thought can transform educators' understanding of how students learn. In M. S. C. Thomas, D. Mareschal, & I. Dumontheil (Eds.), *Educational neuroscience*. Routledge.

Johnson, M., & De Haan, M. (2015). *Developmental cognitive neuroscience: An introduction*. Wiley Blackwell.

Kahneman, D. (2012). *Thinking, fast and slow*. Penguin.

Karpicke, J. D., & Grimaldi, P. J. (2012). Retrieval-based learning: A perspective for enhancing meaningful learning. *Educational Psychology Review*, 24 (3), 401–418. https://doi.org/10.1007/s10648-012-9202-2.

Kelley, P., & Whatson, T. (2013). Making long-term memories in minutes: A spaced learning pattern from memory research in education. *Frontiers in Human Neuroscience*, 7, 589. https://doi.org/10.3389/fnhum.2013.00589.

Kieckhaefer, C., Schilbach, L., & Bzdok, D. (2021). Social belonging: Brain structure and function is linked to membership in sports teams, religious groups and social clubs (preprint). *bioRxiv*. https://doi.org/10.1101/2021. 09.06.459167.

Knowland, V. C. P., & Rogers, C. J. (2021). How neuroscience can help struggling pupils. *TES*. https://www.tes.com/magazine/article/how-neuroscience-can-help-struggling-pupils.

Kontra, C., Lyons, D. J., Fischer, S. M., & Beilock, S. L. (2015). Physical experience enhances science learning. *Psychological Science*, 26 (6), 737–749.

Korol, D. L., & Gold, P. E. (1998). Glucose, memory, and aging. *The American Journal of Clinical Nutrition*, 67 (4), 764S–771S. https://doi.org/10.1093/ajcn/67.4.764S.

Korver, A. M. H., Konings, S., Dekker, F. W., Beers, M., Wever, C. C., Frijns, J. H. M., Oudesluys-Murphy, A. M., & DECIBEL Collaborative Study Group. (2010). Newborn hearing screening vs later hearing screening and developmental outcomes in children with permanent childhood hearing impairment. *JAMA*, 304 (15), 1701–1708. https://doi.org/10.1001/jama.2010.1501.

Kuhl, P. K., Lim, S.-S., Guerriero, S., & van Damme, D. (2019). Developing minds in the digital age: Towards a science of learning for 21st century education. OECD. https://doi.org/10.1787/562a8659-en.

Kurdziel, L., Duclos, K., & Spencer, R. M. C. (2013). Sleep spindles in midday naps enhance learning in preschool children. *Proceedings of the National Academy of Sciences of the United States of America*, 110 (43), 17267–17272. https://doi.org/10.1073/pnas.1306418110.

Lakoff, G., & Johnson, M. (2003). *Metaphors we live by* (new ed.). University of Chicago Press.

Lakoff, G., & Núñez, R. E. (2000). *Where mathematics comes from: How the embodied mind brings mathematics into being* (pp. xvii,493). Basic Books.

Lederbogen, F., Kirsch, P., Haddad, L., Streit, F., Tost, H., Schuch, P., Wüst, S., Pruessner, J. C., Rietschel, M., Deuschle, M., & Meyer-Lindenberg, A. (2011). City living and urban upbringing affect neural social stress processing in humans. *Nature*, 474 (7352), 498–501. https://doi.org/10.1038/nature10190.

Lee, J. J., Wedow, R., Okbay, A., Kong, E., Maghzian, O., Zacher, M., Nguyen-Viet, T. A., Bowers, P., Sidorenko, J., Karlsson Linnér, R., Fontana, M. A., Kundu, T., Lee, C., Li, H., Li, R., Royer, R., Timshel, P. N., Walters, R. K., Willoughby, E. A., … Cesarini, D. (2018). Gene discovery and polygenic prediction from a genome-wide association study of educational attainment in 1.1 million individuals. *Nature Genetics*, 50 (8), 1112–1121. https://doi.org/10.1038/s41588-018-0147-3.

Limb, C. J., & Braun, A. R. (2008). Neural substrates of spontaneous musical performance: An FMRI study of jazz improvisation. *PLoS ONE*, 3 (2), e1679. https://doi.org/10.1371/journal.pone.0001679.

Lloyd-Fox, S., Blasi, A., Volein, A., Everdell, N., Elwell, C. E., & Johnson, M. H. (2009). Social perception in infancy: A near infrared spectroscopy study. *Child Development*, 80 (4), 986–999. https://doi.org/10.1111/j.1467-8624.2009.01312.x.

Lombrozo, T. (2017). Learning by thinking. Edge.org. Available at: https://www.edge.org/conversation/tania_lombrozo-learning-by-thinking.

Luk, G., Bialystok, E., Craik, F. I. M., & Grady, C. L. (2011). Lifelong bilingualism maintains white matter integrity in older adults. *Journal of Neuroscience*, 31 (46), 16808–16813. https://doi.org/10.1523/JNEUROSCI.4563-11.2011.

Maguire, E. A., Gadian, D. G., Johnsrude, I. S., Good, C. D., Ashburner, J., Frackowiak, R. S. J., & Frith, C. D. (2000). Navigation-related structural change in the hippocampi of taxi drivers. *Proceedings of the National Academy of Sciences*, 97 (8), 4398–4403. https://doi.org/10.1073/pnas.070039597.

Martin, N. C., Piek, J., Baynam, G., Levy, F., & Hay, D. (2010). An examination of the relationship between movement problems and four common developmental disorders. *Human Movement Science*, 29 (5), 799–808. https://doi.org/10.1016/j.humov.2009.09.005.

Maslow, A. H. (1943). A theory of human motivation. *Psychological Review*, 50 (4), 370–396. https://doi.org/10.1037/h0054346.

Masson, S., Potvin, P., Riopel, M., & Foisy, L.-M. B. (2014). Differences in brain activation between novices and experts in science during a task involving a common misconception in electricity. *Mind, Brain, and Education*, 8 (1), 44–55. https://doi.org/10.1111/mbe.12043.

McDermott, H., Lane, H., & Alonso, M. (2021). Working smart: The use of 'cognitive enhancers' by UK university students. *Journal of Further and Higher Education*, 45 (2), 270–283. https://doi.org/10.1080/0309877X.2020.1753179.

McMahon, K., Yeh, C. S.-H., & Etchells, P. J. (2019). The impact of a modified initial teacher education on challenging trainees' understanding of neuromyths. *Mind, Brain, and Education*, 13 (4), 288–297. https://doi.org/10.1111/mbe.12219.

Melby-Lervåg, M., & Hulme, C. (2013). Is working memory training effective? A meta-analytic review. *Developmental Psychology*, 49 (2), 270–291. https://doi.org/10.1037/a0028228.

Millar, R. (1991). Why is science hard to learn? *Journal of Computer Assisted Learning*, 7 (2), 66–74. https://doi.org/10.1111/j.1365-2729.1991.tb00229.x.

Mireku, M. O., Barker, M. M., Mutz, J., Dumontheil, I., Thomas, M. S. C., Röösli, M., Elliott, P., & Toledano, M. B. (2019). Night-time screen-based media device use and adolescents' sleep and health-related quality of life. *Environment International*, 124, 66–78. https://doi.org/10.1016/j.envint.2018.11.069.

Moore, D. S. (2013). Current thinking about nature and nurture. In K. Kampourakis (Ed.), *The Philosophy of Biology* (pp. 629–652). Springer.

Nathan, M. J. (2021). *Foundations of embodied learning: A paradigm for education*. Routledge. https://www.routledge.com/Foundations-of-Embodied-Learning-A-Paradigm-for-Education/Nathan/p/book/9780367349769.

Ng, B. (2018). The neuroscience of growth mindset and intrinsic motivation. *Brain Sciences* 8 (2), 20. https://doi.org/10.3390/brainsci8020020.

Nin, A. (1961). *Seduction of the Minotaur*. Swallow Press.

Norton, E. S., Kovelman, I., & Petitto, L.-A. (2007). Are there separate neural systems for spelling? New insights into the role of rules and memory in spelling from functional magnetic resonance imaging. mind, brain and education. *The Official Journal of the International Mind, Brain, and Education Society*, 1 (1), 48–59. https://doi.org/10.1111/j.1751-228X.2007.00005.x.

Oberauer, K. (2019). Working memory and attention: A conceptual analysis and review. *Journal of Cognition*, 2 (1), 36. https://doi.org/10.5334/joc.58.

OECD. (2007). Understanding the brain: The birth of a learning science. OECD. https://doi.org/10.1787/9789264029132-en.

Office for National Statistics. (2018). Deaths by age, sex and underlying cause registrations 2017 for England and Wales. Available at: www.ons.gov.uk/.../birthsdeathsandmarriages/deaths.

Overbye, K., Walhovd, K. B., Paus, T., Fjell, A. M., Huster, R. J., & Tamnes, C. K. (2019). Error processing in the adolescent brain: Age-related differences in electrophysiology, behavioral adaptation, and brain morphology. *Developmental Cognitive Neuroscience*, 38, 100665. https://doi.org/10.1016/j.dcn.2019.100665.

Paivio, A., Walsh, M., & Bons, T. (1994). Concreteness effects on memory: When and why? *Journal of Experimental Psychology: Learning, Memory, and Cognition*, 20 (5), 1196–1204. https://doi.org/10.1037/0278-7393.20.5.1196.

Perry, T., Lea, R., Jørgensen, C. R., Cordingley, P., Shapiro, K., Youdell, D., Harrington, J., Fancourt, A., Crisp, P., Gamble, N., & Pomareda, C. (2021). *Cognitive science in the classroom.* Educational Endowment Foundation, 372.

Peters, S., Atteveldt, N. V., Massonnié, J., & Vogel, S. E. (2020). Everything you and your teachers need to know about the learning brain. *Frontiers for Young Minds.* https://doi.org/10.3389/978-2-88966-026.

Peters, S., & Crone, E. A. (2017). Increased striatal activity in adolescence benefits learning. *Nature Communications*, 8 (1), 1983. https://doi.org/10.1038/s41467-017-02174-z.

Petersen, S. E., & Posner, M. I. (2012). The attention system of the human brain: 20 years after. *Annual Review of Neuroscience*, 35, 73–89. https://doi.org/10.1146/annurev-neuro-062111-150525.

Polderman, T. J., Benyamin, B., De Leeuw, C. A., Sullivan, P. F., Van Bochoven, A., Visscher, P. M., & Posthuma, D. (2015). Meta-analysis of the heritability of human traits based on fifty years of twin studies. *Nature Genetics*, 47 (7), 702–709.

Pope, R., Francis, B., Hamer, M., Hutchinson, J., Lock, S., Moore, R., & Scutt, C. (2019). *Early career framework* (p. 43). Department for Education.

Posner, J., Polanczyk, G. V., & Sonuga-Barke, E. (2020). Attention-deficit hyperactivity disorder. *The Lancet*, 395 (10222), 450–462. https://doi.org/10.1016/S0140-6736(19)33004-1.

Posner, M. I., & Rothbart, M. K. (2014). Attention to learning of school subjects. *Trends in Neuroscience and Education*, 3 (1), 14–17. https://doi.org/10.1016/j.tine.2014.02.003.

Posner, M. I., Rothbart, M. K., Sheese, B. E., & Tang, Y. (2007). The anterior cingulate gyrus and the mechanism of self-regulation. *Cognitive, Affective, & Behavioral Neuroscience*, 7 (4), 391–395. https://doi.org/10.3758/CABN.7.4.391.

Prochiantz, A. (2010). Evolution of the nervous system: A critical evaluation of how genetic changes translate into morphological changes. *Dialogues in Clinical Neuroscience*, 12 (4), 457–462.

Pueyo, T. (2021). You're a neuron. Available at: https://unchartedterritories.tomaspueyo.com/.

Quigley, A., Muijs, D., & Stringer, E. (2018). *Metacognition and self regulated learning.* Education Endowment Foundation.

Rager, K. B. (2009). I feel, therefore, I learn: The role of emotion in self-directed learning. *New Horizons in Adult Education and Human Resource Development*, 23 (2), 22–33. https://doi.org/10.1002/nha3.10336.

Ramani, G. B., & Siegler, R. S. (2008). Promoting broad and stable improvements in low-income children's numerical knowledge through playing number board games. *Child Development*, 79 (2), 375–394. https://doi.org/10.1111/j.1467-8624.2007.01131.x.

Ramani, G. B., & Siegler, R. S. (2011). Reducing the gap in numerical knowledge between low- and middle-income preschoolers. *Journal of Applied Developmental Psychology*, 32 (3), 146–159. https://doi.org/10.1016/j.appdev.2011.02.005.

Rasch, B., & Born, J. (2013). About sleep's role in memory. *Physiological Reviews*, 93 (2), 681–766. https://doi.org/10.1152/physrev.00032.2012.

Rayner, K. (1998). Eye movements in reading and information processing: 20 years of research. *Psychological Bulletin*, 124 (3), 372–422. https://doi.org/10.1037/0033-2909.124.3.372.

Ritchhart, R., Church, M., & Morrison, K. (2011). *Making thinking visible: How to promote engagement, understanding, and independence for all learners*. John Wiley & Sons.

Ritchhart, R., & Perkins, D. (2008). Making thinking visible. *Educational Leadership*, 65 (5), 57–61.

Ritchie, S. J., & Tucker-Drob, E. M. (2018). How much does education improve intelligence? A meta-analysis. *Psychological Science*, 29 (8), 1358–1369. https://doi.org/10.1177/0956797618774253.

Sabbagh, M. A., & Baldwin, D. A. (2001). Learning words from knowledge-able versus ignorant speakers: Links between preschoolers' theory of mind and semantic development. *Child Development*, 72 (4), 1054–1070. https://doi.org/10.1111/1467-8624.00334.

Sarkar, A., Dowker, A., & Kadosh, R. C. (2014). Cognitive enhancement or cognitive cost: Trait-specific outcomes of brain stimulation in the case of mathematics anxiety. *Journal of Neuroscience*, 34 (50), 16605–16610.

Schmied, A., Varma, S., & Dubinsky, J. M. (2021). Acceptability of neuroscientific interventions in education. *Science and Engineering Ethics*, 27 (4), 52. https://doi.org/10.1007/s11948-021-00328-3.

Schwartz, D. L., Tsang, J. M., & Blair, K. P. (2016). *The ABCs of how we learn: 26 scientifically proven approaches, how they work, and when to use them* (pp. xvi,367). W. W. Norton & Co.

Selita, F., & Kovas, Y. (2019). Genes and Gini: What inequality means for heritability. *Journal of Biosocial Science*, 51 (1), 18–47. https://doi.org/10.1017/S0021932017000645.

Senju, A., & Csibra, G. (2008). Gaze following in human infants depends on communicative signals. *Current Biology*, 18 (9), 668–671. https://doi.org/10.1016/j.cub.2008.03.059.

Serrallach, B., Groß, C., Bernhofs, V., Engelmann, D., Benner, J., Gündert, N., Blatow, M., Wengenroth, M., Seitz, A., Brunner, M., Seither, S.,

Parncutt, R., Schneider, P., & Seither-Preisler, A. (2016). Neural bio-markers for dyslexia, ADHD, and ADD in the auditory cortex of children. *Frontiers in Neuroscience*, 10, 324. https://doi.org/10.3389/fnins.2016.00324.

Sharman, R., Illingworth, G., & Harvey, C.-J. (2020). The neuroscience of sleep and its relation to educational outcomes. In M. S. C. Thomas, D. Mareschal, & I. Dumontheil (Eds.), *Educational neuroscience*. Routledge.

Siegler, R. S., & Ramani, G. B. (2008). Playing linear numerical board games promotes low-income children's numerical development. *Developmental Science*, 11 (5), 655–661. https://doi.org/10.1111/j.1467-7687.2008.00714.x.

Siegler, R. S., & Ramani, G. B. (2009). Playing linear number board games—but not circular ones—improves low-income preschoolers' numerical understanding. *Journal of Educational Psychology*, 101 (3), 545–560. https://doi.org/10.1037/a0014239.

Sigman, M., Peña, M., Goldin, A. P., & Ribeiro, S. (2014). Neuroscience and education: Prime time to build the bridge. *Nature Neuroscience*, 17 (4), 497–502. https://doi.org/10.1038/nn.3672.

Simmonds, A. (2014). How neuroscience is affecting education. Wellcome Trust.

Siugzdaite, R., Bathelt, J., Holmes, J., & Astle, D. E. (2020). Transdiagnostic brain mapping in developmental disorders. *Current Biology*, 30 (7), 1245–1257. e4. https://doi.org/10.1016/j.cub.2020.01.078.

Smolen, P., Zhang, Y., & Byrne, J. H. (2016). The right time to learn: Mechanisms and optimization of spaced learning. *Nature Reviews Neuroscience*, 17 (2), 77–88. https://doi.org/10.1038/nrn.2015.18.

Sousa, D. A. (2010). *Mind, brain, & education: Neuroscience implications for the classroom*. Solution Tree Press.

Sousa, D. A. (2011). *How the brain learns* (4th ed.). Corwin.

Soylu, F., Raymond, D., Gutierrez, A., & Newman, S. D. (2017). The differential relationship between finger gnosis, and addition and subtraction: An fMRI study. *Journal of Numerical Cognition*, 3 (3), 694–715.

Standards & Testing Agency. (2011). Year 1 phonics screening check assessment framework (p. 27). *HMSO*. Crown Copyright.

Steele, J., Ferrari, P. F., & Fogassi, L. (2012). From action to language: Comparative perspectives on primate tool use, gesture and the evolution of human language. *Philosophical Transactions of the Royal Society B: Biological Sciences*, 367 (1585), 4–9. https://doi.org/10.1098/rstb.2011.0295.

Sweller, J. (2010). Cognitive load theory: Recent theoretical advances. In J. L. Plass, R. Moreno, & R. Brünken (Eds.), *Cognitive load theory* (pp. 29–47). Cambridge University Press. https://doi.org/10.1017/CBO9780511844744.004.

Temple, E., Deutsch, G. K., Poldrack, R. A., Miller, S. L., Tallal, P., Merzenich, M. M., & Gabrieli, J. D. E. (2003). Neural deficits in children with dyslexia ameliorated by behavioral remediation: Evidence from functional MRI. *Proceedings of the National Academy of Sciences*, 100 (5), 2860–2865. https://doi.org/10.1073/pnas.0030098100.

Thomas, M. S. C. (2019). Response to Dougherty and Robey (2018) on neuroscience and education: Enough bridge metaphors—interdisciplinary research offers the best hope for progress. *Current Directions in Psychological Science*, 28 (4), 337–340. https://doi.org/10.1177/0963721419838252.

Thomas, M. S. C. (2020). Developmental disorders: Few specific disorders and no specific brain regions. *Current Biology*, 30 (7), R304–R306. https://doi.org/10.1016/j.cub.2020.02.019.

Thomas, M. S. C., Ansari, D., & Knowland, V. C. P. (2019). Annual research review: Educational neuroscience: progress and prospects. *Journal of Child Psychology and Psychiatry*, 60 (4), 477–492. https://doi.org/10.1111/jcpp.12973.

Thomas, M. S. C., Knowland, V., & Rogers, C. (2020). *The science of adult literacy*. World Bank Group. https://doi.org/10.1596/33278.

Thomas, M. S. C., Mareschal, D., & Dumontheil, I. (Eds.) (2020). *Educational neuroscience: Development across the life span*. Routledge.

Thomas, M. S. C., & Rogers, C. (2020). Education, the science of learning, and the COVID-19 crisis. *Prospects*, 49 (1–2), 87–90. https://doi.org/10.1007/s11125-020-09468-z.

Thorndike, E. L., & Woodworth, R. S. (1901). The influence of improvement in one mental function upon the efficiency of other functions. II. The estimation of magnitudes. *Psychological Review*, 8 (4), 384–395. https://doi.org/10.1037/h0071280.

Tokuhama-Espinosa, T. (2010). *Mind, brain, and education science: A comprehensive guide to the new brain-based teaching*. W. W. Norton & Co.

Tokuhama-Espinosa, T. (2014). *Making classrooms better: 50 practical applications of mind, brain, and education science*. W. W. Norton & Co.

Tomova, L., Andrews, J. L., & Blakemore, S.-J. (2021). The importance of belonging and the avoidance of social risk taking in adolescence. *Developmental Review*, 61, 100981. https://doi.org/10.1016/j.dr.2021.100981.

Torrijos-Muelas, M., González-Víllora, S., & Bodoque-Osma, A. R. (2021). The persistence of neuromyths in the educational settings: A systematic review. *Frontiers in Psychology*, 11, 3658. https://doi.org/10.3389/fpsyg.2020.591923.

Tulis, M. (2013). Error management behavior in classrooms: Teachers' responses to student mistakes. *Teaching and Teacher Education*, 33, 56–68. https://doi.org/10.1016/j.tate.2013.02.003.

Ullman, S. (2007). Object recognition and segmentation by a fragment-based hierarchy. *Trends in Cognitive Sciences*, 11 (2), 58–64. https://doi.org/10.1016/j.tics.2006.11.009.

UNESCO. (2003). Education in a multilingual world: UNESCO education position paper. UNESCO Digital Library. Available at: https://unesdoc.unesco. org/ark:/48223/pf0000129728.

Valladolid-Acebes, I., Merino, B., Principato, A., Fole, A., Barbas, C., Lorenzo, M. P., García, A., Del Olmo, N., Ruiz-Gayo, M., & Cano, V. (2012). High-fat diets induce changes in hippocampal glutamate metabolism and neuro-transmission. *American Journal of Physiology-Endocrinology and Metabolism*, 302 (4), E396–E402. https://doi.org/10.1152/ajpendo.00343.2011.

Van der Borght, K., Kóbor-Nyakas, D. É., Klauke, K., Eggen, B. J. L., Nyakas, C., Van der Zee, E. A., & Meerlo, P. (2009). Physical exercise leads to rapid adaptations in hippocampal vasculature: Temporal dynamics and relationship to cell proliferation and neurogenesis. *Hippocampus*, 19 (10), 928–936. https://doi.org/10.1002/hipo.20545.

Van Elk, M., van Schie, H. T., Hunnius, S., Vesper, C., & Bekkering, H. (2008). You'll never crawl alone: Neurophysiological evidence for experi-ence-dependent motor resonance in infancy. *NeuroImage*, 43 (4), 808–814. https://doi.org/10.1016/j.NeuroImage.2008.07.057.

Varela, F. J., Rosch, E., & Thompson, E. (1991). *The embodied mind: Cognitive science and human experience*. MIT Press.

Vasilopoulos, F., & Ellefson, M. R. (2021). Investigation of the associations between physical activity, self-regulation and educational outcomes in childhood. *PLoS ONE*, 16 (5), e0250984. https://doi.org/10.1371/journal.pone.0250984.

Walter, J., & Hümpel, A. (2017). Introduction to epigenetics. In R. Heil, S. B. Seitz, H. König, & J. Robienski (Eds.), *Epigenetics: Ethical, legal and social aspects* (pp. 11–29). Springer Fachmedien. https://doi.org/10.1007/978-3-658-14460-9_2.

Walton, G. M., & Cohen, G. L. (2011). A brief social-belonging intervention improves academic and health outcomes of minority students. *Science*, 331 (6023), 1447–1451.

Wang, Y., Hong, S., & Tai, C. (2019). China's efforts to lead the way in AI start in its classrooms. *Wall Street Journal*. https://www.wsj.com/articles/chinas-efforts-to-lead-the-way-in-ai-start-in-its-classrooms-11571958181.

Whitebread, D., Bingham, S., Grau, V., Pasternak, D. P., & Sangster, C. (2007). Development of metacognition and self-regulated learning in young children: Role of collaborative and peer-assisted learning. *Journal of Cognitive Education and Psychology*, 6 (3), 433–455. https://doi.org/10.1891/194589507787382043.

Whitebread, D., Coltman, P., Pasternak, D. P., Sangster, C., Grau, V., Bing-ham, S., Almeqdad, Q., & Demetriou, D. (2009). The development of two observational tools for assessing metacognition and self-regulated learning in young children. *Metacognition and Learning*, 4 (1), 63–85. https://doi.org/10.1007/s11409-008-9033-1.

Whitebread, D., & Neale, D. (2020). Metacognition in early child development. *Translational Issues in Psychological Science*, 6 (1), 8–14. https://doi.org/10.1037/tps0000223.

Whiting, S. B., Wass, S. V., Green, S., & Thomas, M. S. C. (2021). Stress and learning in pupils: Neuroscience evidence and its relevance for teachers. *Mind, Brain, and Education*, 15 (2), 177–188. https://doi.org/10.1111/mbe.12282.

Wilhelm, I., Diekelmann, S., & Born, J. (2008). Sleep in children improves memory performance on declarative but not procedural tasks. *Learning & Memory*, 15 (5), 373–377. https://doi.org/10.1101/lm.803708.

Wilson, D., & Conyers, M. (2020). *Five big ideas for effective teaching: Connecting mind, brain, and education research to classroom practice.* Teachers College Press.

Woodworth, R. S., & Thorndike, E. L. (1901). The influence of improvement in one mental function upon the efficiency of other functions (I). *Psychological Review*, 8 (3), 247–261. https://doi.org/10.1037/h0074898.

Yan, V. X., Eglington, L. G., & Garcia, M. A. (2020). Learning better, learning more: The benefits of expanded retrieval practice. *Journal of Applied Research in Memory and Cognition*, 9 (2), 204–214. https://doi.org/10.1016/j.jarmac.2020.03.002.

Yeager, D. S., Carroll, J. M., Buontempo, J., Cimpian, A., Woody, S., Crosnoe, R., Muller, C., Murray, J., Mhatre, P., Kersting, N., Hulleman, C., Kudym, M., Murphy, M., Duckworth, A. L., Walton, G. M., & Dweck, C. S. (2022). Teacher mindsets help explain where a growth-mindset intervention does and doesn't work. *Psychological Science*, 33 (1), 18–32. https://doi.org/10.1177/09567976211028984.

INDEX

Please note that page references to Figures will be in **bold**, while references to Tables are in *italics*. Footnotes will be denoted by the letter 'n' and Note number following the page number.